"I've watched Mary Beth Albright eat, and I flourish in her career over the last decade. A true authority on all things food, her book is a departure from the expected and does a world of good through one of our most important places: the dinner table."

—Bobby Flay, chef

"Food has an incredible power to heal bodies and nourish minds, to connect and repair communities, to feed the few and the many. In *Eat & Flourish*, Mary Beth Albright makes the compelling case that by understanding food holistically, we can unlock its potential to improve our physical and emotional well-being."

—José Andrés, chef

"As a chef, nutrition and nourishment is at the forefront of what I do. Mary Beth Albright presents an impressive exploration of the interconnectivity of these elements—and beyond—in *Eat & Flourish*. It is an outstanding and comprehensive book for today's food and health enthusiast."

—Thomas Keller, chef/proprietor, The French Laundry

"A fun and illuminating look at how food affects mental health . . . [Albright's] gift for making science accessible and entertaining is on full display. . . . The research is eye-opening, and Albright's genial tone makes her an ideal tour guide. The result is a first-rate program for eating better."

—*Publishers Weekly*, Starred Review

"A brilliant exploration of the connection between food and emotional well-being . . . *Eat and Flourish* is a compelling and practical guide to how small changes in daily diets might make someone feel their best. Among the countless books extolling the virtues of 'healthy' eating, this stands apart because of Albright's focus not just on nutrients but also on the 'circle of food, nutrients, pleasure, and connection.' *Eat and Flourish* presents a more intentional way of eating that supports every aspect of how a person feels—physically, mentally, and emotionally. And in a world that's rife with chaos, the privilege of being intentional about what and why we eat is not one to be taken lightly."

—Kerry McHugh for Shelf Awareness, Starred Review

Eat & Flourish

Eat & Flourish

HOW FOOD SUPPORTS
EMOTIONAL WELL-BEING

Mary Beth Albright

Countryman Press

An Imprint of W. W. Norton & Company
Independent Publishers Since 1923

Copyright © 2024, 2023 by Mary Beth Albright

All rights reserved
Printed in the United States of America

Illustrations on pages iii, vii: B.illustrations/Shutterstock.com; pages 23, 66, 93, 103, 106, 111, 142, 155: @ Alhontess/iStockphoto.com; pages 109, 151, 161, 165: @ Epine_art/iStockphoto.com

For information about permission to reproduce selections from this book, write to Permissions, Countryman Press, 500 Fifth Avenue, New York, NY 10110

For information about special discounts for bulk purchases, please contact W. W. Norton Special Sales at specialsales@wwnorton.com or 800-233-4830

Manufacturing by Lakeside Book Company
Book design by Marysarah Quinn
Production manager: Devon Zahn

Library of Congress Cataloging-in-Publication Data

Names: Albright, Mary Beth, author.
Title: Eat & flourish : how food supports emotional well-being / Mary Beth Albright.
Other titles: Eat and flourish
Description: First edition. | New York : Countryman Press, an imprint of W. W. Norton & Company, Independent Publishers Since 1923, [2023] | Includes bibliographical references and index.
Identifiers: LCCN 2022028999 | ISBN 9781682686904 (hardcover) | ISBN 9781682686911 (epub)
Subjects: LCSH: Nutrition. | Food—Psychological aspects. | Well-being.
Classification: LCC TX353 .A465 2023 | DDC 612.3—dc23/eng/20220803
LC record available at https://lccn.loc.gov/2022028999

978-1-68268-903-5 pbk.

Countryman Press
www.countrymanpress.com

An imprint of W. W. Norton & Company, Inc.
500 Fifth Avenue, New York, NY 10110
www.wwnorton.com

10 9 8 7 6 5 4 3 2 1

FOR MY SISTERS:

Ann, who taught me that art and beauty are everywhere.

Evelyn, who taught me the power of good mental health.

Contents

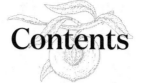

Eat & Flourish

Foreword

AS A CHEF AND A PHYSICIAN, I have been standing at the intersection of food and well-being for more than 30 years. Until recently it has been a fairly lonely corner, but thankfully that is changing. In the past decade, armed with mounting evidence that food and cooking can improve all aspects of health. I started a Culinary Medicine program, first at the Tulane School of Medicine and now at George Washington University School of Medicine and Health Sciences. This coursework, which has been adopted by universities across the nation, helps teach the benefits of nutrition-related lifestyle changes, such as cooking. In my quest to teach and use the important connection between well-being and food, I've been fortunate to meet amazing chefs, health care professionals, policy makers, researchers, and journalists who care deeply about great food as an important component of well-being.

One of those journalists whom I met a few years back immediately impressed me as caring not just about this topic but also about her craft. She is the author of the book you are now reading: Mary Beth Albright. Mary Beth and I met when she interviewed me for a profile about culinary medicine that she was writing for *National Geographic*. It was clear that she had done her homework and had established a solid foundation of knowledge about the subject. She delivered a terrific description of the state of the art at the time.

She delivers again with this book.

Food research has come a long, long way in the four decades that I have been involved in the nutrition world. This is the challenge that you, the reader, faces: science evolves, and that means changes in recommendations around food and health.

People are understandably confused because in one decade we are told to substitute margarine for butter, and a decade later we're told that margarine has actually been contributing to health issues. The good news is that we now have a much more solid understanding of how what we eat can both harm us and benefit us.

It can sometimes be hard to know what to believe. This book is one that you can trust and one you can believe. It is a solid review of the science and provides direct, day-to-day application for your life and your health by showing the impact of one of the most important aspects of living longer and living well: how food supports your emotional well-being.

Most of us think of diets or eating plans or nutrition as applying to the usual suspects, such as heart attacks, strokes, diabetes, hypertension, and high cholesterol. However, the same healthy food principles apply to our moods, emotions, pleasure, energy, and mental health.

Mary Beth does an amazing job in leading us through the complex neurologic anatomy and hormone responses. Trust me, understanding neurotransmitters, endocrine responses, gamma-aminobutyric acid, dopamine, adrenocorticotropic hormone, and cortisol activity is tough stuff even for health care professionals. Mary Beth makes understanding things such as the amygdala and hippocampus easy and even fun—and both of those brain structures are just fun to say out loud.

This is because she has translated the hard stuff in a way that allows her to lead readers through the impact that food has on everything—from sights and sounds to pleasure and socialization (to name only a few stops on the journey she takes us on). That trip starts with a tour of the body itself, and she acts as the consummate tour guide, offering a complete picture of how what we eat impacts the various organ systems that contribute to and modulate our moods, energy, and emotions.

That grand tour continues and ends up spanning the world, literally. We are transported to the Monell Chemical Senses Center in Philadelphia; the Mind-Body Institute in Australia; a functional magnetic resonance imaging center in Oregon; a microbiome lab in Ireland; farms in Ashburn, Virginia, and in outer space (yes, outer space); a longevity center at Stanford; the Japanese Ministry of Health; and the Mediterranean to understand how following an old-world diet can have a tremendous impact on how food makes us feel.

As a tour guide of our bodies and of the world of research, she continues to ground the information in the important fact that eating is an intimate and personal social event that is critical to our well-being.

In the first five chapters, you are going to go on a journey that will establish a foundation and convince you through solid evidence that there is a direct connection between what you consume and how you feel. That alone makes for a fantastic book, but the bonus is Chapter 6: an equally solid four-week plan that will help you use the evidence presented in the first five chapters to transform your kitchen, your menus, and your mood.

As the corner of food and health research becomes more and more crowded, I am really proud to have journalists and authors like Mary Beth Albright standing with us. Quality work always shines, and this book is one that can help transform the quality of your life.

Eat well, eat healthy, enjoy life!

Timothy S. Harlan, MD, FACP, CCMS
Associate Professor of Medicine, George Washington
University School of Medicine and Health Sciences
President, Culinary Medicine Specialist Board
Editor-in-Chief, *Health meets Food: The Culinary Medicine
Curriculum,* CulinaryMedicine.org

Introduction

Food is pleasurable. We feel joy when we eat, whether it's a juicy peach, crusty bread, or chocolate—and we especially feel uplifted when we're sharing that pleasure with other people. This emotional reaction also shows up physically via brain activity that can be mapped and studied. Sex, great music, and delicious food all activate the same circuitry that lights up to tell you: This feels good.

All of the above is just some of what I learned when I found myself lying down inside a tube, motionless, drinking milkshakes, kale juice, and wine through straws while half a dozen scientists watched.

Depending on what I ate, the functional MRI (fMRI) scanning my brain showed varying degrees of pleasure parties in my head. As I reviewed the images later, I could literally see how eating, something I do a few (OK, maybe several) times each day, influences how I experience the world. And if my food choices affect my brain activity so acutely in the moment, then surely there are long-lasting changes too.

That brain scan was just part of the larger story about how food can improve our emotional well-being. The brain and gut send signals back and forth that affect decisions, relationships, satisfaction, and mental health.

Those signals depend a lot on the kind and quality of food we eat, and the latest science shows that certain foods are particularly beneficial.

This book is about the art and science of what and how to eat for emotional well-being—that is, how we react to life's inevitable everyday ups and downs, pressures, and changing relationships. Let's dig in and discover how we can eat and flourish in everyday life.

—————

THE LINK BETWEEN food and mood has been brewing for more than two decades. In 2006, I was leaving my office at the surgeon general's headquarters when a medical journal passed my desk. One article in *The International Review of Psychiatry* in particular caught my attention: It was about food. But instead of focusing on the connection between our eating habits and physical health, or addressing specific conditions like obesity, heart disease, high cholesterol, or diabetes, it was about how food can moderate our responses to stress.

This study showed that eating omega-3 fatty acids showed "considerable promise in preventing aggression and hostility." Being deficient in omega-3 may result in lower levels of serotonin, the study noted, and lower serotonin levels are linked to mood disorders. Pills designed to increase serotonin have been available by prescription for decades. (Pills I have personally benefited from, as Ina Garten would say, store-bought is fine!)

The researcher behind that 2006 study, Joseph Hibbeln, had also found in 1998 that more fish consumption was associated with lower depression risk. Hibbeln wasn't some nutty wellness guru; he worked at the National Institutes of Health and was a commissioned officer of the United States Public Health Service. I thought to myself that, if the government accepts that nutrition could be mainstream medicine for mental health, this could be the beginning of a food-mood revolution.

By the time I started my current job as a writer and editor at the *Washington Post* years later, I had kept up with the trickle (and then deluge) of new peer-reviewed science documenting how what we eat affects mental health. The research going into this question is extensive and complex. It considers how emotions affect both what we eat and how we eat, and how those two things interact with our bodies to determine the value (calories, nutrients, and mood-supporting chemicals, among others) we pull from our food for our mental health.

Now we can see plenty of peer-reviewed, measurable results about the food–emotional well-being connection, such as:

» Depressed young men with poor diets had a significant reduction in symptoms over 12 weeks when they followed a Mediterranean diet;

» People who eat 2 cups of produce daily had lower stress levels than those who ate less than 1 cup;

» Stressed people who had high levels of omega-3 fatty acids had less anxiety and inflammation than stressed people who did not;

» Eating an inflammatory diet is associated with a 25 percent greater risk of depression and an 85 percent increase in emotional distress, and anti-inflammatory foods (foods that calm inflammation) are linked to better mental health outcomes;

» When mice exhibiting healthy behaviors received the gut microbes (which are highly influenced by diet) of mice exhibiting anxiety, the healthy mice start acting anxiously; and

» The more people eat with others, the happier and more satisfied they are with their lives.

The phrase "emotional eating" has a negative connotation, as we've conflated it with binge eating or mindless eating—think tearing through bags of salty chips or pints of ice cream—which brings brief relief but also problems in the long term. But there are a lot of definitions of emotional eating, and with the right foods we can reclaim this biological reality as something that supports us. We can get rid of the shame associated with our various hungers and sources of pleasure. Emotional eating and well-being are not opposites. They are pieces of the same whole. The question isn't how to forget about emotional eating; our biology has made sure that we can never do that. The question is how we can use our emotional eating for our long-term well-being. In the following pages, we will look at the latest research in neuroscience, nutrition, and even microbiology, and apply those insights to real life.

In my life I've found it critical to have practical steps alongside groundbreaking information, so I've been developing recipes ever since I began writing about food. The success of my recipes even gave me the opportunity to devote a year of my life to being a finalist on *The Next Food Network Star*—an experience that was not great for my mental health, but that's another story entirely. In this book, each chapter ends with a simple recipe designed for you to live deliciously, simply, and with your well-being as a top priority.

A healthy relationship with food is about more than just looking at nutrients, and eating for mental health is more than swapping out candy bars for beans. In my research journey, I wanted to consider the science of both nutrition and pleasure, as well as what insights neuroscience can offer with respect to both the nutrients in our food and how we cook it. I wanted to look at food's transformational power to gather, to soothe, to please. I wanted scientific rigor and information from the top scientists doing the most cutting-edge research worldwide in the many scientific disciplines that cover food.

This was personal, too. I was proud of surviving big personal challenges over the years: family-of-origin issues, career changes, divorce. I've lived a fortunate life; I've also experienced tragedy (see, you really can have it all). How could I start living my priorities daily through food: maintaining a sustainable mood, dealing with my emotions, and rediscovering an uninhibited joy in cooking and eating?

I looked at research that would answer questions I thought would help me and possibly others:

> » How does food affect emotions?
> » How does food affect emotional health?
> » How do emotions affect our food choices?

» How do emotions affect our nutritional needs?
» Which science is reliable and which is just hype?
» Can cooking (or stress baking) really make you feel better?

The questions—and, as I found, the answers—are all inextricably linked with each other in a circle of food, nutrients, pleasure, and connection. Food is an integral part of the body, a mash-up of raw materials and experiences that we choose every day. It's a Möbius strip that has no beginning or end, and I explored it in the context of how we can use food to support emotional health.

As I kept reading studies and journal articles from different fields of science, I discovered it's not just *what* we eat, it's *how* we eat that affects mental health. Everything about food and cooking—selecting what to eat, choosing the best ingredients, smelling meals cooking in our homes, working with our hands, remembering feelings tied to certain flavors, communing with people around the dining table—is an opportunity to improve mood and help process emotions.

Eating is a relatively low-cost and low-risk intervention that can be added to many other forms of mental health care. And especially these days, it's important to remember that you don't have to be in a mental health crisis to benefit from mental health care. Science shows that consistent attention to our mental health can, in some cases, prevent or alleviate crises.

We can use food to improve our minds and, in turn, use our minds to improve our food experiences. Just as food influences the substances our bodies make that affect our brains, our brains affect the amount of pleasure we get out of food. It's a cycle that goes around and around, with food affecting our bodies and our bodies affecting our food choices.

Armed with knowledge, we can use the food-mood connection to create a virtuous (rather than vicious) cycle and actually enjoy ourselves along the way. Life is too short, and too long, to not exploit the power of the food-mood connection.

Science shows that eating well isn't about being perfect (thank goodness because the pursuit of perfection can be a real downer). It's about establishing eating patterns that consider how the brain and the body talk to each other; your food impacts what kind of conversation they have. You can feel good about your food *and* get pleasure from it.

Mental health is more than the absence of mental illness. Food can be a source of real, lasting joy. Let's look at how to harness that.

CHAPTER 1

Emotional Eating

"To eat is a necessity, but to eat intelligently is an art."
—FRANÇOIS DE LA ROCHEFOUCAULD

COMFORT AND FOOD go hand in hand for us humans, but until recently, researchers had no idea why. Is it our memories, nostalgia, mouthfeel, connecting with people? Is it distraction, pleasure, trying to correct a nutrient deficiency? Everyone has their favorite comforting food experiences and is intimately familiar with the healing power of a meal, whether it's a convivial feast with friends or eating a steaming bowl of stew solo while watching movies on a snowy Sunday.

There are things about food that seem like magic but are actually just wonderful aspects of reality. A feeling of love for someone motivates us to cook vegetable soup, that vegetable soup creates immediate pleasure and emotions of happiness, then the vegetables turn into chemical reactions in the body that support the long-term ability to manage the emotional triggers that happen in everyone's lives. How we look at food is ultimately a window into ourselves and our personal life histories: how we choose, how we take care of ourselves, how we relate to others.

We are discovering a lot about how each individual body uses food. Some bodies pull lots of critical nutrients out of food; some bodies have less capacity to process and absorb what they need. Some bodies have good bacteria living inside of them that support production of neurotransmitters, such as serotonin and gamma-aminobutyric acid (GABA), both known for mental health benefits. (The allure of neurotransmitter production is so powerful that in 2022 a company announced they had developed the first GABA-enhanced tomato.) Some bodies need help getting more of those good gut bacteria. Some bodies have a highly sensitive and reactive brain reward system for food. Deriving a greater reward from something means we will seek it out more frequently because our minds and bodies are built for pleasure; we have evolved to seek it, receive it, and, whenever possible, increase it. And with newly discovered science, we can use our good human brains to think just a little more broadly than using food only for immediate pleasure. Then we can harness the ancient biological power of our bodies for long-term well-being.

Each of the hundreds of studies I read about food and emotional well-being, on its own, provided valuable information in its specific field of scientific research. But when you put them all together, cross disciplines and national boundaries, there is a clear picture of steps we can take to improve our emotional and mental health through food. Some of it has to do with what we eat; some of it has to do with how we eat, which for a while was a casualty of our obsession with superfoods and functional foods. Superfoods, a colloquial term for foods that pack in more nutrients per calorie than other foods, do exist. But nutrient-dense foods are just part of the story, a piece of the puzzle rather than the whole picture. Most of us can't even keep nutrient differences straight in our own heads, let alone make food choices based on them. A lot of us focus on the paradigm of having an occasional superfood to do penance for eating junk the rest of the time, but science shows that a strong whole-foods eating pattern is the best way to deal with emotional health and can help our bodies deal much better with occasional junk food. In the last chapter of this book, you'll find some practical tips about applying all this science in your everyday life.

Your food choices impact your emotional state. This occurs both immediately, as you get pleasure from eating, and over the long term, as the food you eat is the foundation of the chemicals your body makes, from neurotransmitters like dopamine and serotonin to hormones like adrenaline and cortisol.

And your emotional state impacts your food choices. This biology belongs to everyone, supermodels and sumo wrestlers alike. (I hope someday there is a sumo wrestler-supermodel.) I know that many Silicon Valley innovators claim that food is just fuel and wish they never had to stop working to eat, but even meal replacement drinks come in different flavors. Even when we don't leave our keyboards, we still would maybe rather taste strawberry than chocolate in our protein shakes.

Your emotions, and how you act on them, are processed by your nervous system. Different emotions have different physical reactions, many of which you're not aware of, that create differing physical needs. And your nervous system—the body's communication system, which has the brain at its helm—is fueled by food.

It's a loop, and no one knows which came first:

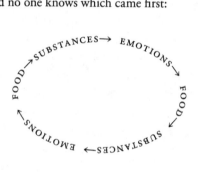

We'll examine specific foods that help with the physical effects of different emotions and the science behind the emotional effects of food. But first, let's look at where emotions come from—which, maybe not coincidentally, is also where our perception of flavor comes from: the nervous system.

The Nervous System

The nervous system is based on highly specialized cells called neurons. Most cells in the human body are rounded. But neurons look as if they have lots of tangles of tiny roots coming off them. They reach out to other neurons to transfer information all over the body. Neurons are concentrated in the brain but are located all throughout the body, including a very active collection residing throughout your digestive system. Neurons send signals to each other at hundreds of miles per hour, so we perceive stimuli—such as the physical sensation of putting your hand on a hot stove—as pretty much immediate. Thanks to neurons, the nervous system relays communications throughout your body quicker than the blink of an eye.

Neurons get used to patterns of communication pathways. When you do something repeatedly, the neurons change their connections to "learn" how to meet more easily and quickly. So sometimes your neurons see a pattern and think, *oh, I know this,* and then follow a series of familiar connections. But we've recently discovered that you can change these patterns and grow new paths of neuron connections based on your behavior (including the food you eat), an idea called neuroplasticity.

To survive, we need to know what is happening in the external world. This is where our senses come in: smell, taste, touch, sight, hearing. The neurons all over our bodies transfer that sensory information about what's happening to our brains. Our brains decide how we feel about the stimuli—a reaction known as emotions. Emotions create reactions in our bodies, causing us to behave according to how we feel about what's happening around us. You may see a fire and have the emotion of fear, which makes physical adjustments in your body to respond to the stimuli that caused the fear, preparing you to run from danger. Or you could see a fire and have the emotion of joy because it's in a fireplace, which makes your body relax.

STIMULI → EMOTIONS → ACTIONS

Neurons are concentrated in the brain, the organ at the top of the central nervous system (CNS) that gathers and processes information and sends signals to the rest of the body. (The CNS consists of the brain and the spinal cord.) Neurons help process stimuli, contributing to how we feel and, ultimately, to our actions. This makes a lot of sense when we think about the stimuli that we are aware of in everyday life. Your boss might be grumpy, which creates an emotion in you, and you choose how to act in response to it. Someone is laughing and staring at you, which creates an emotion, and you choose how to act in response to it. It may have something to do with you, or it may be that they're laughing at something else and their eyes just gazed at you briefly.

But the thing is, we are not always aware of the stimuli. The body's neurons are constantly communicating to the brain what's happening in every part of the body.

One way neurons communicate with each other is through passing chemicals, called neurotransmitters, both to other neurons and sometimes to other types of body cells that aren't neurons. These chemical releases are triggered by electrical impulses from any kind of stimuli—what we read or see or hear or even think. You're doing it right now. This sentence is a stimulus. It's causing electrical impulses in your brain that send neurotransmitters between neurons. The sense of smell (which we'll examine in more detail later) takes molecules in the air—stimulus—and connects those molecules with neurons in our noses that detect smell. Then the brain identifies what particular odor we're smelling and how we feel about it.

The nervous system runs alongside another body communication system that uses the bloodstream as its method of travel: the endocrine system. Chemical messengers that travel through the bloodstream are called hormones. Hormones are secreted by glands throughout the body. And, because the brain controls the glands, the nervous system and the endocrine system are connected. The endocrine system communicates more slowly than the nervous system because the hormones have to travel through blood to get to other cells, and blood is a slower method of transportation than messages leaping directly from neuron to neuron. The lines between the systems of communication can get fuzzy—for example, some scientists consider serotonin, important for mental health, both a hormone and a neurotransmitter.

BRAIN STRUCTURE FOR NON-SCIENTISTS

Learning about the brain can feel overwhelming to a non-scientist. When my kid was in preschool, they learned about their emotions through something called the "hand model of the brain."

First, make a fist with your thumb tucked inside.

Your fist represents a brain when it's well. Your thumb represents the limbic (primal) regions of the brain, the amygdala and hippocampus, which are bundles of neurons shaped like an almond and a seahorse, respectively. The amygdala (almond) governs instinct, and the hippocampus (seahorse) controls emotional memory recall.

So generally the stimuli are filtered through both your past experiences and your instincts to inform your feeling about what's happening. The limbic system also includes the hypothalamus, which regulates appetite, weight, and body temperature.

These almond- and seahorse-shaped bits of gray matter are where information from our senses is dumped and sorted. These are the caveman parts of the brain. Personally, my limbic system is drama, drama, drama all the time from past trauma that informs my current instincts. I have to work to make sure my actions do not automatically match the drama. You do not want the primal regions of your brain running your life unhinged and uncontrolled. You have to pair the limbic with a healthy and functioning logical brain.

That's where the cortex comes in. The four fingers over your thumb in our closed-fist model represent the cerebral cortex, or the "thinking brain." This is the upper part of the brain and includes the prefrontal cortex. This is where logic and reason live, where we can decide whether the fear that our primitive brain senses is a real threat. When you look at your fist, you can see that your thinking brain—the four fingers—"hugs" the primal brain, positioned to tell that jumpy caveman area that it's safe when it senses fear. But that's only if your cerebral cortex is functioning well.

When the cerebral cortex is overloaded with information, you may "flip your lid." My then-four-year-old son's teachers showed this to their students by releasing the four fingers (the thinking brain goes off the rails), sending them straight up in the air, leaving the thumb (the primal brain) no longer hugged. The caveman brain is exposed and running the show.

I find a couple of other kid-centered explanations of the brain compelling. As has happened forever in history, science and popular culture collide. In the video game *Bloodborne*, one fictitious evil character is named

Amygdala and it lives in the Nightmare Frontier. It looks like a human-sized, haunting neuron, a terrifying spiderlike creature with a brain for a head. I also love the character Man-Thing from Marvel Comics. He used to be a man but now is a swamp beast with no rational thinking. He just stumbles around, sensing the emotions of others around him and being intensely affected by them. Essentially, he's a highly sensitive person (or, I guess, a highly sensitive thing). When he is around emotions like anger or fear, he reacts by secreting a corrosive acid that burns other people. He eats his own waste, so this walking reactive emotion beast becomes a freestanding ecosystem. When others feel fear, he can't help them—he just burns them. Importantly, Man-Thing can burn even other superheroes. His emotions are powerful.

This all sounds very familiar. Perhaps you know someone like this. Perhaps you *are* someone like this. Thankfully, it is possible to turn distress intolerance into resilience and emotional agility. We don't have to bang around the world as a self-contained ecosystem, destroying everything in our wake when we are faced with difficult emotions. Let's take a look at how the feeling of fear works in the nervous system.

Let's go back to the fire example: Say there is a fire somewhere in your home. Burning materials release molecules into the air. Those molecules reach your olfactory neurons, which perceive an odor. The amygdala jumps to attention to start the fear process. The cortex then applies logic to the fear. Maybe you remember that earlier you lit a lovely fire in the hearth, so everything is fine. Or maybe there is no explanation other than there is a dangerous fire in the house and you need energy to fight it.

When the amygdala is activated, it tells another part of the limbic system, the hypothalamus, to tell the pituitary gland to make hormones that will help the body react to fear, particularly a chemical called adrenocorticotropic hormone (ACTH). The pituitary gland shoots these hormones out into the bloodstream. One effect of all that ACTH is that your body releases cortisol, which raises blood sugar, heart rate, and white blood cells (which fight infection)—in other words, it increases the available resources in your body to react to the threat that caused your fear.

Meanwhile, your nervous system tells your adrenal glands to pump out another hormone, epinephrine, otherwise known as adrenaline. It's the same stuff you find in epi pens to inject into someone having an allergic reaction. Epinephrine relaxes the muscles in the airways to allow more air to come in with each breath (so that when you're afraid, you can run away faster) and tightens blood vessels (sending more blood to your veins, which go to your organs, so you can act quickly). Adrenaline also raises heart rate and increases blood flow to your brain and muscles, and it raises blood sugar levels.

I'm simplifying and condensing the many processes that happen inside the human body, but the substances our body pumps out directly relate to our well-being. There is debate over whether hormonal state by itself is necessary or sufficient to cause mental health issues in humans. Mental health is complicated and involves many factors, but on a broad physical level, depression is often associated with a lack of dopamine and serotonin. Stress is an excess of norepinephrine and epinephrine. Happiness is a lot of serotonin and sometimes dopamine. And all these substances—and our emotions—are affected by the food that we eat.

Problems arise in today's world when we don't use—or sometimes even need—those resources made available to us through stress. Modern threats like traffic jams, watching disturbing news, or having an awful boss are unavoidable but don't always require (and in fact are often made worse by) fleeing or fighting. So all those hormones, all those downstream effects of fear, are just floating around your body, gearing you up for a physical fight that never happens. Your nervous system is all pumped up with nowhere to go. And the more you have these natural reactions to these modern stressors, the more ingrained they become. There is a theory of brain plasticity called Hebb's postulate which, simplified, is known as "cells that fire together wire together." When a cell is consistently activated at the same time as another cell, those cells learn to work together. The bond between them strengthens. So if we can work on ways to get cells to fire together differently, the brain—with its plasticity—can change the pathways that neurons use. Hebb's postulate reminds me that every day we are teaching our neurons how to fire together.

There are lots of ways to calm the nervous system—deep breathing, mindfulness, yoga, exercise—and I recommend all of these. And food, both cooking it and eating it, can help calm the nervous system from many directions.

Ozempic

No matter what your opinion of injectable weight-loss drugs, such as Ozempic, the new information we have from them is invaluable, both physically and socially.

Patients report that taking this class of medications reduces the "food noise" in their own heads. They can look at a plate of cookies and not be consumed with thoughts of whether they should eat one, whereas, before Ozempic, the cookies would spur a person's internal dialogue weighing the pros and cons of whether the cookie would be delicious enough to be "worth it" at the cost of a larger body. The internal dialogue is, at least in part, due to diet culture.

"Diet culture" wasn't a phenomenon people talked about when I was growing up in the 1980s and 1990s—there was just a general overall understanding that if you had a larger body, there was something wrong with you. There are many definitions of "diet culture," but the one that speaks to me the most recognizes that the diet culture discussion is wholly different from nutrition science. Diet culture is insidious because it uses valid nutrition science to give people an invalid message that their choices are wrong and, therefore, something is wrong with them.

The best definition I've heard of diet culture is the idea that there is a moral hierarchy of food choices and body sizes and types. If a fat woman eats ice cream in a bathing suit, it is inherently more wrong and reprehensible than a thin woman eating ice cream in a bathing suit.

However, there is no morality inherent to food choices. There is morality involved in how we treat humans, animals, and the planet, but these aren't specific to food choices. We know that higher consumption of ultra-processed foods is linked to lower emotional well-being, but there is nothing morally deficient in someone choosing ultra-processed foods, particularly because food choices involve many complicated factors. People with PTSD, for example, show changes in their gut microbiomes that may make adherence to a Mediterranean-type diet with fewer ultra-processed foods more difficult.

A 2023 report from UCLA found that people who are exposed to racial or ethnic discrimination may be more susceptible to food-related health problems because of a stress response that alters the brain's reaction to food reward and decision-making. When participants were shown food cues—juicy burgers or creamy ice cream—those with more discrimination experiences had greater brain activation in areas that regulate cravings and appetite. The same activation did not occur when participants were shown foods like vegetables. There were also noted changes in the gut microbiomes of participants who had experienced discrimination, with potential dysregulation of the gut-brain messaging pathways. Research like this may have been dismissed in the past before we had people's anecdotal experience with Ozempic and hard data on weight loss that comes with it.

The new class of weight-loss drugs seems to intercept the way we think about highly palatable foods, and patients instead seek out some whole-food alternatives. This has caused a ripple effect in the food industry among businesses that make more money when you buy more food. Walmart released a statement that states customers on Ozempic buy less food. The investment banking firm Morgan Stanley conducted a survey that showed that people on weight-loss injectables reduce calories by 20 to 30 percent, and most of the respondents said they mostly cut back on sugar. The fast-food company Chipotle has said it expects its sales to rise as people on weight-loss drugs choose whole foods, which its menu is based on, rather than the fried foods of many fast-food companies. Other food companies, such as Nestlé, have announced that they're working on creating new products directly targeting people using drugs like Ozempic. So weight-loss "companion products" could be the next big thing in the food industry.

One company creates highly palatable ultra-processed food that is convenient and easy to store and eat—this addresses the real problem that customers don't have the time, knowledge, or inclination to cook as much.

A different company develops a drug to help you stop wanting that quick and tasty food—another real problem. Yet another company creates products to have alongside the drug; there is a tail-swallowing-snake feeling to this cycle. Eating whole foods for pleasure is a simple but not easy solution.

Diet culture is why you would rather have someone see you eating a carrot instead of Cheetos, that there is some virtue associated with the vegetables and something demonic about ultra-processed foods. Diet culture leads to shame, to people eating "bad" foods in secret, a bifurcation of our food reality and what we want others to believe is our food reality.

Preliminary but mounting research shows that this class of drugs may be useful for brain-based diagnoses, such as Parkinson's and Alzheimer's, and other conditions associated with addiction and impulsiveness, such as alcoholism. Earlier weight-loss interventions, such as gastric bypass surgery, often resulted in patients shifting obsessive thoughts from food to something else—sex, for example, or smoking. Food was no longer an option because of a physically smaller stomach, so the brain turned elsewhere.

These drugs are able to address something happening in the brain that mediates food choices. Medicine and media have been talking about obesity as a disease for decades, but the diet culture remnants have continuously perpetuated the idea that there is something morally wrong with people who take in more calories—they are hedonistic, indulgent—when eating ultra-processed foods may just be a survival mechanism for dealing with stress for particularly susceptible brains.

This moment opens up a whole new anti-diet culture dialogue: if drugs can address obesity, then maybe there isn't something morally wrong with people who have larger bodies. Maybe the quick judgments we make about people's character based on their body types and food choices aren't accurate at all. And maybe beating ourselves up over our own food choices is in fact the exact opposite of what we should be doing; we should be showing ourselves and others compassion. Maybe our emotional well-being and the emotional well-being of others is precisely what we should be working on when it comes to food, and that means practicing kindness.

Of course, lowering stress is often an unaffordable luxury. Working multiple jobs, coping with budgets in an age of inflation, or living in an under-resourced neighborhood can all be unrelenting sources of stress—they're upstream problems. Addressing upstream problems can take time and large-scale intervention. Equipping ourselves with the knowledge to feed ourselves as we want to be fed can be a downstream solution.

Emotions

Emotions are a valuable, if messy, tool for living an authentic life. Emotions are a superpower, a sign of strength. They allow you to take in large amounts of information; your body then processes that information to tell you how you feel about it. The outside world affects our brains, our brain creates emotions, and emotions affect our bodies. Food fuels this entire process. It's a cycle, and it can be vicious or virtuous, depending in part on your food choices.

Stress comes from feeling overwhelmed by events or emotions. The event that we react to can be something that we perceive as being a problem, even if it's not. Everyone has experienced walking by a group of people who started whispering and worried that they're whispering about us, even when we have no idea what they're saying—that can be a stressor. We all want to get rid of that tense, tight feeling that comes with stress.

There is compelling science that your body needs more of certain nutrients when you're in certain emotional states—more magnesium when you're stressed, for example, and zinc when you're sad—which we will discuss more specifically later. But it can be harder to make those food choices when you're in an intensely negative emotional state. Research shows that people feeling intensely negative emotions were more likely to make health-supporting food choices *if* they think the negative feelings are fleeting. And other evidence shows that the ability to come out of a negative emotional state is likelier if you make certain food choices. Again, we see that the food-emotion cycle can be vicious or virtuous, but it remains a cycle.

Think of it in terms of sleep. When you're well rested, your baseline mood is often higher than if you're exhausted. And then imagine someone cuts you off in traffic. How mad do you get? If you've had sleep and your baseline mood is good, you're less likely to get mad or take it personally, and further less likely to have reactions to that anger that are not in your best interest. If you've had less sleep, it can cause longer-lasting or more intense anger and lead to actions that aren't in your best interest.

Our past experiences, including trauma, can significantly inform how we interpret the sensory information we receive from the outside world. We can't do anything to change our past experiences. But we can understand that, in the moment of having an emotion, that emotion may be a response to something that happened to us years ago and might have nothing to do with the present situation.

But the answer isn't to cut ourselves off from emotions, even if they're unpleasant. In studies, decreased emotional expression leads to a decrease in positive emotions and poor psychological adjustment. Heart rate can increase when we are suppressing emotions too. When emotions are numbed, they aren't available to us to learn more about ourselves and create a better life. It's short-term survival at the expense of long-term progress and wellness—tempting at first, particularly if you have a drama-drama-drama limbic system, but a bad deal in the end.

We'll get into specific emotions and how, if left unacknowledged, they can damage our mental health in Chapter 5. Throughout the book we'll be looking at how our food choices impact both our emotions and how we act on our emotions.

HANGER

I found other personal food experiences are backed by science: "Hanger" is real, for example. "Hangry" is a portmanteau of "hungry" and "angry"; in 2018, it was added to the Oxford English Dictionary. Recently, researchers identified activity in neurons in the brain's hypothalamus, the ancient region of the limbic system that coordinates both hunger and emotion. Not having enough food activates these brain cells, known as AgRP neurons, in mice. The neurons signal both hunger and, at the same time, a negative feeling.

"Hangry neurons" is the name researchers have informally given AgRP neurons. Think about a time when you skipped breakfast and later snapped at a colleague in a meeting. Or those times when you wait too long between lunch and dinner, and a late-afternoon crash leads to a low-energy scavenging for quick-energy food. Regulating hangry neuron activity can change behavior, including eating behavior, in mice. When we look at rodents' brain activity while they're eating, we can see that active hangry neurons create two effects, feeling awful *and* eating voraciously, until the neurons are no longer activated. Then the bad feelings go away. Chronic stress causes changes in hangry neurons, which is not really surprising considering that the hypothalamus, where the hangry neurons live, is not protected from toxins in the blood by what we call the "blood-brain barrier," which we will learn more about when we discuss inflammation. As a result, all the toxic effects of stress can travel straight from our blood to the hypothalamus.

There is a theory about why the body evolved so that hunger is associated with anger. It goes like this: During evolution, when food was scarce, it was critically important to have the extra motivation of anger—in addition to hunger—to go seek food. Feelings of hunger might not have been enough to alert us to the urgency of eating to our evolution. Today, we think of the bad feelings that come with hunger as just part of hunger—but AgRP researchers believe that we just perceive them as the same because they happen together. Scientists believe that getting food was so important that the body developed anger and hunger as double motivation to eat, and this may be how these hangry neurons may have evolved.

In our modern world, where food is everywhere and sugary, high-fat, calorie-dense foods that are highly palatable can be the most accessible and least expensive choice, hangry neurons are not crucial for our survival. They may actually cause us to overeat. We still have them, though, another potential mismatch between how we evolved and how we live now. Some people feel hanger more than others, which may mean that your ancestors had the kinds of powerful AgRP neurons that drove them to survive. (Kind of makes me have a little more respect for hanger.)

At the Monell Chemical Senses Center in Philadelphia, Dr. Amber Alhadeff's lab studies hangry neurons, feeding behavior, and how gut-brain communication influences what we eat. The invasive technology required to research how hangry neurons react in real time while a subject is eating means that research showing the activity in these specific neurons has all been conducted in animal subjects thus far. In Alhadeff's studies, when the stomach gets food, it tells the brain almost instantaneously that there is no need to be angry anymore. When food is introduced, the neurons immediately calm down and simultaneously stop sending both hunger and negativity signals. Hungry and angry feelings disappear at the same time as food calms the hangry neurons. But when hangry neurons are exposed to chronic, unpredictable stress, it can lead to despair and inability to enjoy activities. And that stress can make food an even more rewarding prospect to our brains.

This may all sound rather obvious. But, evolutionarily, being hungry didn't have to go hand in hand with negative emotions. We could have just had a hungry signal that told us "find food now," but instead we evolved to have a negative feeling along with that feeling of hunger that is doubly, intensely motivating.

As Alhadeff explains, from her lab's research, "We've discovered that you really need that gut signaling to have long reductions, sustained reductions in AgRP activity. And this is important because it means if you have a Diet Coke, you get that taste in your mouth and maybe your neurons will transiently inhibit, but that activity will come right back up. Your hunger levels will come right back up. And so, in the absence of that gut signaling, you really don't shut off these hangry neurons." There is also some very recent evidence that AgRP neurons may contribute to depression, although we don't yet understand how.

A 2023 study found hunger hormones produced in the gut influence decision-making in the brain of mice. The hippocampus, which is critical for decision-making and using memories to guide future behavior to act in our best interest, has less activity when the hunger hormone ghrelin is in the blood. The amount of ghrelin is inversely proportional to how actively the hippocampus is used. When researchers forced activity in the hippocampus in hungry mice by blocking the effects of ghrelin on the hippocampus, the mice stopped eating—even though the mice had not ingested any food.

As the researchers put it, hormones "contextualize" the feeling of hunger for the brain. When there is a lack of food and ghrelin, the brain says "eat"—a signal that has served humanity well in our evolution. When there is a lack of food and no ghrelin, the brain does not necessarily say "eat." This may have been devastating for evolution, but interfering with our own bodies' brilliant messaging system may seem a compelling method of decreasing our consumption of the very ultra-processed food that may be confusing signals in the first place.

Hunger, emotions, and behavior are all mixed up in the same highly specialized brain cells. And those brain cells are directly connected to your digestive system, which is directly influenced by what and how you eat.

Four Snacks to Buy at a Convenience Store

Because sometimes you need to eat right now and you didn't pack a little baggie of snacks because you have a real life and just didn't get to it.

1. **Nuts:** Dry roasted is best because there is no added oil (which is often industrially processed oil).
2. **Raisins:** They are densely packed with sugar but a little can go a long way, particularly when added to other snacks like nuts and seeds.
3. **Seeds:** Sunflower seeds with the shell on can be their own ritual—cracking off the shells and popping the meaty kernel into your mouth.
4. **Popcorn:** Fiber, crunch, childhood nostalgia—I can't say enough good things about popcorn.

Nutritional Psychiatry

"At the time, people thought I was a bit mad," Felice Jacka, now a co-director of the Food and Mood Centre in Australia and the president of the International Society for Nutritional Psychiatry Research, told me, referring to her PhD thesis on food and mental health in 2009. But Jacka was seeing pieces of evidence that people's diets were related to their experience of and risk for depression and anxiety. There was Hibbeln's omega-3 work.

There was a mouse study showing diet can stimulate the growth of new neurons in the hippocampus. Another study showed that improving and diversifying food in prison populations significantly reduced incidents of violence; it was titled "Crime and Nourishment."

Jacka's paper associated Western-style diets—high in sugar and unhealthful fats, low in nutrients, high in ultra-processed foods—with depression and anxiety in women. Although she was just a PhD candidate, her thesis was published as a cover article in the *American Journal of Psychiatry* in 2010.

Around the same time on the other side of the world, stress neurobiologist John Cryan had his eureka moment. Neurobiologists generally focus on the brain, but his fellow researchers in Ireland were showing that the brain wasn't necessarily the starting point for regulating the body's stress response. He conducted a study in 2009 that showed, as he expected, that animals who were stressed in early life and experienced early trauma developed symptoms of psychiatric disorders later in life. The surprise was that these traumatized mice also developed gut problems, such as irritable bowel syndrome, alongside their mental disorders.

So Cryan tested their gut microbiomes—the community of trillions of microorganisms (tiny life forms that we can see only through microscopes) that help with digestion—and found that traumatized animals had different compositions of their gut microbiomes. What we eat greatly affects the gut microbiome and whether we have helpful or harmful bacteria living inside of us. We'll dig into the many factors influencing the gut microbiome in Chapter 3, but Cryan wondered: If the microorganisms inside us help with digestion and if stress affects our microbiomes, then emotional states could influence what the body does with food and how food could influence our emotional states.

Cryan next turned to whether we can target the gut to deal effectively with stress. His later research showed that when his lab introduced beneficial bacteria into the animals' digestive systems, their anxious and depressive behavior dampened equal to or more than the effect of the antidepressant escitalopram (Lexapro). Antidepressants and food together could have an even greater effect.

Spin the globe over to Japan around the same time. A Japanese study showed that "germ-free" animals who are specially bred not to have any microbes inside of them, thus no gut microbiome, have an increased stress response, further associating stress regulation with the microbes inside of us. And the microbes inside us are, in turn, affected by the food we eat.

In 2013 a study showed that feeding junk food to mice damages the mouse hippocampus; after four days, the mice showed decreased cognitive functions related to the hippocampus (the seahorse), which interacts with the amygdala (the almond) in the limbic system. Cryan and others started coming up with research protocols that could show the effect in humans along with more in-depth animal studies.

Cryan brought in a small sample of healthy human volunteers to do stressful tasks like public speaking or difficult arithmetic. Those who ate the bacteria *Bifidobacterium longum* (found in yogurt) exhibited less stress during traditionally stressful tasks versus those who didn't. Jacka's group published a study showing that the Western diet is associated with a smaller hippocampus.

Then, in 2017, Jacka published peer-reviewed results of the first human intervention specifically targeting and measuring the effect of diet on humans' mental health. Known as the SMILES trial, this was a psychiatric epidemiology study showing that dietary intervention alone impacted mood.

SMILES was the first randomized, controlled study to ask: If we change the diet of people with clinical depression, does it impact their mental health? The answer was yes.

Relative to some studies, the sample size was small and the duration was short because of the difficulties inherent in dietary research. Diet studies are difficult because, short of watching participants' every move or putting a camera on someone's head and recording everything they eat and do all day every day, diet studies depend on people recalling and recording what they eat. Jacka wanted to do a longer and more intensive study, but human nutrition epidemiological studies can be expensive and require the most unpredictable of subjects—humans—making shorter studies more reliable than longer ones. But SMILES's importance is reflected in that it remains one of the most-cited studies about the food-mood connection.

Jacka's lab divided 67 people with depression symptoms into two groups: one that received support with a counselor and one that received dietary support from a dietitian to make small changes to transfer to a Mediterranean-style diet. (In an ideal world, of course, we all would have both—but this study was measuring the effects of one versus the effects of the other.)

The Mediterranean diet has a long and culturally rich history based on the eating habits of people who live around the Mediterranean Sea—Italy, Spain, Greece, and Turkey. In dietary trials, the Mediterranean diet is defined by specific foods—whole grains, seafood, nuts, beans, fruits, olive oil, and vegetables.

One-third of participants in the Mediterranean diet group saw their depression symptoms go into remission. And the more the subjects adhered to a Mediterranean-style diet, the more remission they experienced. Plus, important for equal access, the food the diet-intervention participants ate was about 20 percent less expensive than the diet that they had eaten prior to the study.

This study showed that lower-cost prevention and treatment interventions for two huge health issues—poor diet and mental health—could actually address each other. It contributed to global interest and the explosion of research done since. SMILES inspired subsequent larger and more specific studies that support the conclusion that what we eat affects how we feel. In a 2022 study of 72 young men (aged 18 to 25) with moderate to severe depression and poor diet, 30 percent of participants had failed to respond to standard treatments for depression, such as medication. As mentioned briefly in the Introduction, switching to the Mediterranean diet for 12 weeks brought a significant improvement in their symptoms of depression. And participants expressed interest in continuing to eat a Mediterranean diet after the study ended—as we all know, getting excited about permanent diet changes is at least half the battle.

In 2020, Cryan's group published a study that included a typically chronically stressed group: university students. Researchers examined psychological and biological changes in students over exam periods and found that students who ate *Bifidobacterium longum* didn't have as many sleep problems. We don't know what the bacteria was doing or precisely how it was doing it, but it was happening.

To be sure, skeptics remain, particularly in the specialty that Cryan himself is a member of. "Neuroscientists tend to look only at the neck upward," he told me. "There is an idea that everything that doesn't have a known mechanism for a causal link—diet is a prime target—should be relegated to the world of complementary and alternative medicine." In other words: It can't hurt, but it shouldn't be one of the first things you look to for an intervention. Causal links are difficult for studies about things as complex as emotions and interventions that have wide-ranging effects, such as food.

But because we all have emotions and we all eat, the information is actionable. "There are fundamentals that are true for everyone," Jacka says. "You may need to tweak based on individual markers," but there is enough evidence that there are dietary truths for most humans, truths we will dive into in the following chapters.

Now we have solid evidence that food affects the body everywhere, including from the neck up, and that eating for mental health is about an eating pattern. The more you follow a mentally healthy eating pattern, studies show, the more your body can handle occasional deviations from that pattern.

It then follows that we can turn what we may see as our biggest weakness—food—into our greatest strength. And we can do it in a pleasurable way. It's one thing to know the science; it can be quite another to incorporate it faithfully into real life. Because it's no use having an eating pattern that supports the nutrients we need for emotional health if we have so little pleasure that it damages our emotional well-being.

Savory Breakfast Muffins

Even the most mindful of us need a fast breakfast sometimes. These muffins have everything required from a great quick breakfast. They're compact, have protein and starch baked in, and are delicious. You can make the muffins in advance and keep them in the fridge for a quick grab and go. Plus getting produce, especially vegetables, first thing in the morning is always a win.

MAKES 6 MUFFINS

1 tablespoon olive oil
½ medium onion, finely chopped
1 small garlic clove, minced
1 cup halved cherry tomatoes
3 eggs, beaten
1 cup cooked quinoa
1 cup grated aged Gruyère cheese (optional, and can substitute
    any hard cheese you love)
1 tablespoon fresh thyme leaves
½ teaspoon kosher salt

Heat oven to 350°F and grease a muffin tin.

Heat oil in a skillet over medium heat and sauté the onion, garlic, and tomatoes until onions are soft and tomatoes are light brown and caramelized, 5 to 7 minutes. Set aside to cool slightly.

In a large bowl, combine the remaining ingredients and the onion mixture and combine.

Pour into the muffin tin and bake for 15 to 20 minutes, until the eggs are set.

Option: Use mini muffin tins for a one-bite, high-protein, and high-fiber breakfast. Just store muffins in the fridge, microwave a couple of mini muffins for 10 seconds, and you're out the door.

CHAPTER 2

Pleasure

"What we learn with pleasure we never forget."
—CHARLES ALFRED MERCIER

Y OU CAN BE A PERSON who loves both eating for health and getting
pleasure from food. It's not an either/or proposition.

Pleasure is a big part of emotional well-being, but it's also often neglected
when we think about eating for health. Pleasure is as much a part of our
physical bodies and as much a necessity as the vitamins and polyphenols
we'll discuss later. Telling people to stay away from pleasurable food is like
teaching only abstinence as sex ed. It's not effective and, if followed to the
letter, it would have humanity-destroying side effects.

Pleasure is a big part of eating. So how do we meet in the middle, to
have smart pleasures that support health?

By embracing the biological basis of pleasure rather than fighting it,
you will better understand a big part of your brain's motivation and use it
to make choices that are in your long-term best interest.

I can't say this enough (and the science supports it): Enjoying your food
is really important.

When we encounter stimuli surrounding food (choosing ingredients,
cooking, eating), the senses send signals to the brain, which decides how
we feel about the stimuli. Everything about food and cooking—smelling
food cooking in our homes, working with our hands, remembering

feelings tied to flavors, communing with people—is an opportunity to improve mood and help process emotions. Working with food is working with your senses.

In the conversations I had with dozens of researchers about the science of emotional eating, they discussed how humans can combine the powerful, biologically based draw of immediate pleasure with the goal of long-term health. There's plenty of immediate, intense pleasure to be had through health-damaging ultra-processed food, food that has been engineered to give tons of pleasure so we will purchase it again. Our work is to use our senses to make whole foods pleasurable to our brains. Some studies showing that potential include:

» A study found that people who regularly followed eating rituals, such as saying grace or preparing food in a certain way they enjoyed, over five days chose more health-promoting food. Enjoyment further increased when the study's subjects performed the ritual themselves, more than if they watched someone else do it.

» A study found that self-preparation of food (cooking) increases people's enjoyment of health-promoting food.

» A 2020 meta-analysis of 77 studies worldwide found that gardening and growing food helps decrease anxiety and depression, improve sleep, and improve cognitive functioning. Gardening is also linked with greater consumption of produce overall.

How Brains Experience Pleasure

After reading dozens of studies about food and pleasure, I wanted to find out more about how, practically, we can use the science to solidify long-term better eating patterns for emotional wellness . . . which brings me back to drinking wine in the fMRI machine.

Dr. Eric Stice is a psychologist and researcher at Stanford University, studying how our brains—and specifically our brains' pleasure centers—respond to food. According to Stice's research, our eating patterns, as in what we eat on a regular basis, can increase the amount of pleasure we get from different foods.

Stice feeds people milkshakes in fMRIs to see how ice cream affects our brain activity, so of course I flew across the country to visit him. FMRIs allow researchers to track brain activity while the subject is doing something to see which parts of the brain get lots of blood rushing to them, for instance, because of the task being performed. This research is a way of seeing parts of the brain light up while it's functioning, all so we can learn more about how brain cells craft our emotional experience of the world. If you're doing something pleasurable, the pleasure centers light up; if you're experiencing sadness, those centers light up.

I was definitely interested in how my brain responds to milkshakes. But I also wanted to know what my brain would do, in comparison, on wine (which I drink fairly often). And how would a milkshake and wine compare with something I don't consume on a regular basis? So I wound up on Stice's doorstep with a bottle of Cabernet and 16 ounces of kale juice, asking to take a spin through his fMRI. He provided the milkshake.

FMRIs have been the basis of a lot of brain research over the past couple of decades, but the technique has its limitations. Specifically, you have to lie perfectly still while you're doing the activity or you won't get readable results. Also, the noise of the machine is so loud they provide earplugs. So I spent more than an hour on my back, very still, inside a tight tube while a specially fitted fMRI straw (attached to a mouthpiece) dripped milkshakes, wine, or kale juice onto my tongue. The straw was connected to reservoirs of liquid outside the fMRI and my "dose" was controlled by the researchers watching me. At the same time, the researchers flashed images of what I was drinking in front of my eyes to see how differently my brain was activated by expecting the different liquids.

The milkshake photo was one of those tall, old-timey glasses with a load of whipped cream and a cherry. It was chocolate and very frosty, and I was supposed to imagine eating a milkshake when I saw it. So I did, envisioning sipping out of the straw, with frozen creaminess hitting and then melting on my tongue. Same with the glass of wine, toasty and tannic, and the kale juice, chilled and brightly bitter. Everything tasted as I expected. But the scans showed that my brain anticipated the wine and milkshake way more, that I was highly alert to my expectations.

I really wanted wine and milkshakes, but when I actually got sips my brain was like, *oh yeah, wine again*—high expectation, not high pleasure. It reminded me of the studies that show that more money doesn't make rich people happier. I still enjoyed the amazing things—ice cream! wine!— that I have had many times before. But they didn't meet my remembered expectations of the tremendous pleasure bomb I received before because my brain had become used to it. This is why, when we frequently eat these foods, we build what Stice calls a tolerance to food.

"We just have one set of reward circuitry in our brains. And what's activated by food, alcohol, drugs—it's the same circuitry," Stice told me. "Anything that makes you feel good, your body will become oriented to remembering the cues that came along with it. It turns out that if you eat more when you're anxious or depressed, these emotional experiences become cues to eat more."

He also found that ultra-processed foods change how our brains function. The same neuroplasticity that benefits us by creating new neurons and forming new neural connections can also be used to humans' detriment by changing our palates through our brains.

Ultra-processed foods tend to hit the pleasure centers of the brain fast and hard. This is because many ultra-processed foods give our brains something that doesn't occur in nature: foods that are high in both fat and sugar (even foods that don't taste sweet to us can sometimes contain a lot of sugar) as well as being extremely easy to find and eat. They're portable and shelf-stable too, so we can have them anywhere. The invention of ultra-processed foods—and these foods have increasingly dominated grocery stores for more than 50 years—can change how our brains operate and influence what our brains find pleasurable.

In one study, Stice examined 100 volunteers, half of whom ate ice cream regularly. The other half rarely or never ate ice cream. In those who rarely or never ate ice cream, the shakes lit up their brains' reward centers—there was lots of pleasure shown in brain activity. The infrequency of eating ice cream meant that when they did choose to eat ice cream, they got intense pleasure hits. Having ice cream once in a while increases the pleasure you get from it.

In those who eat ice cream regularly, there was high anticipation for the ice cream (like my brain scan for wine) but a diminished response when the food was actually being eaten. Still, because of that initial hit of pleasurable anticipation, your brain will again and again crave fast, easy, fat- and sugar-rich calories. These foods can wreak havoc on our moods by increasing inflammation (more on inflammation and mood later), starving our gut microbes, and depriving us of nutrients we need for emotional well-being. We don't know whether we ever reexperience the initial level of pleasure when we eat large quantities of ultra-processed foods for a long time, but we do know we can damage our emotional health while we do it.

Stice's research is particularly interesting when combined with other food studies. For instance, a 2015 study showed that people with mild depression symptoms are more likely to engage in unconsciously eating fatty foods. When we do this, we teach ourselves to associate sadness with foods that don't emotionally support us because of the intense pleasure they bring in the moment. And we can unlearn it too, thanks to neuroplasticity.

Photos of cheesy, juicy hamburgers oozing sauce, or loads of ice cream dripping with caramel and piled high with whipped cream—there's a reason we call it food "porn." When we even just see cues about foods that our brains have associated with high pleasure, dopamine is released. Because dopamine is experienced as a reward, people who eat lots of ultra-processed food become more aware of ultra-processed foods for the next dopamine hit. If I eat a lot of fast-food fries and you eat none and we drive by a fast-food restaurant, I am way more likely to notice the restaurant than you are. And noticing that food is available can be an easy first step to actually eating it. So the more we eat ultra-processed food, the more we just notice it, even when we're not consciously looking for it (even if we just ate and aren't hungry at all).

The more you eat donuts, the more donut cues you notice but the less pleasure your brain gets from actually eating donuts. A white paper bag that donuts come in, or a donut shop or anything that's associated with donuts will make you think of donuts. But then you go to eat the donuts and they don't give as much pleasure as your brain remembers. So you eat more donuts in pursuit of that pleasure, sort of like food pleasure nostalgia.

Stice and other researchers are working on ways to reduce our vigilance to ultra-processed food cues and increase our association of health-supporting foods with pleasure. They've had some success with computer programs and apps that give a negative association with overeating trigger foods. When you see an image of an ultra-processed food you love, for example, the program also shows images of the potential negative effects of that food, such as a fatty liver. Conversely, programs also show good, positive associations with health-supporting foods, such as a smiling person with lettuce. In their research, when subjects used the app, they made better food choices.

Stice's goal is to help us get more pleasure out of foods that we don't necessarily link with pleasure, foods that aren't the high-fat, high-sugar reward bombs. Flavor is conditional on our brains, so it's complicated.

"That's in the nature of working on the neural basis of pleasure," Kent Berridge, a professor and researcher at the University of Michigan, told me. "Pleasure itself is a squishy concept because there are different things that can give you pleasure and different amounts of pleasure and different intensities. Scientists like something in which we can control the variables and come up with something specific."

It's a difficult area, but research protocols are getting creative. In one study, researchers gave drinks to fans after a hockey game. They were all given the same drink, but fans rated the drink sweeter if their team won and more bitter if their team lost. Another study showed that depression levels of subjects affected taste ratings, with depressed people expressing a preference for sugar and experiencing greater intensity of sweet and bitter flavors when having symptoms. Additionally, when people with depression saw happy or sad movie clips, their ability to identify fat in food was blunted by emotions. The authors concluded that emotions "may foster unconscious eating of fatty foods" in depressed people.

To further complicate matters, what we taste one day can be very different than what we taste the next. "Human taste in normal healthy subjects is plastic," states one study in which researchers found that altering serotonin and noradrenaline levels was linked with people identifying food as especially sweet or bitter. The study found that "general anxiety level is directly related to taste perception."

Emotional eating is not a character flaw; it's part of our shared humanity. Even if you're eating Pringles in your car and your hand gets stuck like a monkey trying to get its fist out and refusing to let go of the chip even though it's the only way to get your hand free. Sometimes eating that one last Pringle in the can is a particular kind of pleasure, like licking a plate; lapping up the last of something sticky off hard, cool porcelain; catching the delicious last streaks of, say, caramelized sugar.

At cocktail parties, food writers get asked about the best meal of our lives the same way doctors get asked about whether this mole looks OK. It's a standard question, and when I get it, I describe a meal I ate surrounded by friends while we all sat in rocking chairs on a blue-sky day overlooking the Great Smoky Mountains. We ate barbecue and drank fresh-pressed apple cider while a bluegrass band played Johnny Cash's "Ring of Fire." It was magical. I also sometimes recall a Vermont sugaring off dinner, which celebrates the maple syrup harvest. The sugar shack (where maple sap is boiled and turned into syrup) served as a makeshift kitchen for a chef who incorporated hints of syrup and complementary flavors into each dish while hungry diners snuggled deep into fluffy blankets. Memories of maple glazed salmon still tease me to this day.

Then I turn it on the questioner to see what their favorite meal experience has been. The descriptions always include the food they ate, of course, as does mine. But their answers, too, invariably include atmosphere—where they were, who they were with, sometimes the music that was playing. Pleasure comes from things ancillary to just putting food in your mouth, chewing, and swallowing.

COMFORT FOOD

When I was deep into researching food and pleasure, I went to the source, the woman who is credited by the Oxford English Dictionary with the first publication of the phrase "comfort food," Phyllis Richman. For decades Richman was the restaurant critic at the *Washington Post* and, according to *Newsweek*, the most feared woman in Washington.

Back in 2015, I interviewed her on stage at the Smithsonian for an event on the history of American food criticism. She started as a critic in the mid-1970s and always went in disguise and under a false name. Richman told me a story of one time she went to a formal restaurant and was told her reservation would not be honored because they did not allow ladies wearing pants. So she took her pants off. She happened to be wearing a kind of long tunic shirt, so she just went into the bathroom, took off her pants, popped them in her purse, and went to lunch. If you know this story, you know Phyllis Richman.

Anyway, when I contacted her about the dictionary crediting her with the first use of a much-beloved phrase, she said, "I thought that was pretty exciting; I didn't believe it but I'm happy to accept it." She had a few interesting observations about comfort food.

"Comfort food is really the cornerstone of any region's cuisine," she said. And that's pretty amazing because no matter what nook of the earth you're from, there are comfort foods. "In some areas, comfort food would have no pepper in it. In other areas it would depend on pepper or peppers, such as the Caribbean or mountainous areas of China."

In other words, some parts of comfort food are cultural. I once went to an exhibit during the World's Fair in Milan showing different meals ready to eat (MREs) that different countries' militaries provide for soldiers and how they had evolved through the decades, reflecting how comfort food is both culture- and time-specific. In American MREs today there may be beef stew or peanut butter and jelly spreads. France may supply a cassoulet (a lush casserole of beans and meats) and a little piece of pâté. Italian soldiers get tuna packed in oil and pasta with beans.

Because both flavor and pleasure happen in the brain, all the experiences and expectations we bring to the table—including our nation's dietary tastes in comfort food—affect how we enjoy food. From the moment you interact with your food, whether you are searching for recipes, or visiting a market, or chopping ingredients, or hearing the sizzle in the pan, or seeing a finished dish brought to your plate—your brain brings all these experiences to the table. In this way, food shopping and cooking lead to better food not just because of the stand-alone quality of ingredients but because of the perception we have that the ingredients are of higher quality because we hand-selected them.

Under the heading of "great work if you can get it" is pleasure researcher. Neuroscientist Morten Kringelbach of the University of Oxford is not necessarily what you expect the picture next to "pleasure researcher" in the dictionary to look like. A buttoned-up Danish-born scientist, he looks more like a helpful bookstore clerk. But his research center is called Hedonic Research Group. With the same tone as he might recommend rereading your favorite Jane Austen novel, he conversationally mentions how brain mechanisms generate pleasure, such as an orgasm, that can be seen in fMRIs. Of his appointment at Oxford he says, "Something like sex is very difficult to get any studies done in the UK; we're supposed to close our eyes and think of England. But when they have a Dutch collaborator, you can suddenly start to see what happens when people have orgasms in a brain scanner."

Maybe "orgasm research subject" is the real "great work if you can get it."

Kringelbach and I talked about the tactile pleasure of a Nordic sauna, going from the heat into the snow and back into the heat again. Nordic countries have specific words for this kind of pleasure—uitwaaien ("wind therapy") in the Netherlands and friluftsliv (embracing outdoor life regardless of weather) in Norway. I mention to him that I'm a member of the Diplomatic Sauna Society, a group of people in government, politics, and media who go to the giant sauna in the basement of the Finnish embassy in DC and then run around in the cold. In a professional American setting, though, we don't get naked. "Well, it doesn't count if you don't get naked," Kringelbach insists.

Remember that your brain has one set of pleasure/reward circuitry. His area of research—like Stice's and Berridge's—is what happens in our brains' pleasure rooms. How do parts of the body work together to produce pleasure? Is food pleasure different from other pleasures? Can we ever have too much pleasure?

"Exactly the same things happen in your brain when you have good sex, hear good music, or eat good food," Kringelbach told me. The pleasure that you get from a great meal goes through the same brain patterns as great sex.

Pleasure is Kringelbach's passion. He makes brain computer models that attempt to predict what kind of pleasure you will get from different activities or stimuli. Regardless of the type of activity or stimuli, "it's the same circuitry that underlies all these experiences, the same kind of machine room that has to work, and when it's not working, you suffer from something called anhedonia, the lack of pleasure. We kind of know that the machine room is there at birth—newborn babies exposed to sugar water will lick their lips. And then, how quickly the babies lick is proportional to how sweet the sugar water is." More sugar, faster licking.

When I ask Kringelbach what motivates him to do this kind of research, he gets more philosophical than I expect a scientist to be. "I consider how to think about hedonia—that's Aristotle's word for pleasure—in terms of eudaemonia, which is meaningful engagement in life. Eudaemonia is human flourishing."

To illustrate the effect of pleasure on flourishing, Kringelbach invokes one of his favorite novels and movies, *Babette's Feast*. The plot goes like this: In the 1800s there is a small community of likable people who have denied themselves pleasure for religious reasons. They're less a radical cult, more simple living. One night they are morally obligated to eat an expensive, lush, and very French meal at a banquet. It transforms them and, at least for one evening, they are laughing, playful, and connected with each other in a way they have never experienced. Pleasure changes people, Kringelbach says.

Well-being through food occurs through both sensory qualities of consuming the food and food acting as a gateway to other people.

"When it comes to food," Kringelbach says, "the most important pleasure of all is who you're eating with and the social interactions that come with food."

Have some sympathy for your poor evolving brain. We are born with a pleasure system that responds to sugar. There's nothing we can do about that. Ultra-processed food can, over time, alter the pleasure system's response and therefore reduce the effectiveness of the food in bringing pleasure. The more sugar we eat, the more our brains get used to it and the less likely it is to be rewarding. But at the same time, our brains become more likely to tell us we want sweets when we see a cue about them. That's a tough pattern.

"Food has been manufactured to cheat our brains," Kringelbach opines. "There are companies spending time trying to figure out how to add enough sugar so that we become addicted to these foods. But there are no shortcuts to deep, meaningful engagement, not just with the food but with the people around us as we make and eat the food. And if we don't do that, a kind of anhedonia [inability to feel pleasure] surfaces and we see the kinds of worries people now have about food."

It's a relief to hear a scientist explain this modern phenomenon, to know that there isn't something inherently wrong with us when we suddenly see the bottom of a bowl of ice cream and don't quite remember how we got there. It's still fundamentally human to grow used to and expect pleasure, according to Kringelbach.

Similarly, at researcher Berridge's lab, rats exposed to both sugar and cocaine will typically take lots of both—"I'll have some sugar, I'll have some cocaine, why not?" as Berridge says. They naturally will go to cocaine and sugar equally. But through his research, Berridge can produce a rat that wants sugar over cocaine, or cocaine over sugar, depending on brain manipulation. Some rats develop "an irresistible fascination and attraction" to things that bring them pain, as long as their brains' hedonic hot spots are activated.

Unsurprisingly I discovered during the course of my interviews that Kringelbach and Berridge are friends, and Berridge had the same thesis advisor as Alhadeff, who studies hangry neurons.

So, how can we use this information to increase food pleasure? It starts with the beginning—getting food.

Getting Food

If you want to know whether being in touch with getting your food is essential for well-being, look to the one place that needs to pare everything down to its bare minimum while prioritizing connecting people with their food: outer space.

Space organizations are seriously concerned with food as one of the few ways that astronauts can stay in touch with their own humanity in an environment that is thrilling yet devoid of normal human touch points. Group meals are common every day on the International Space Station to combat the negative effects of isolation.

"It's a custom that the astronauts tend to schedule their meals together," Dr. Gioia Massa of NASA told me. NASA's food lab offers more than 250 culturally appropriate dishes for astronauts, including warm cookies and samosas, all tailored to space travelers' individual tastes and memories of home. Italian astronaut Samantha Cristoferetti even received an espresso maker from the Italian Space Agency.

NASA has a highly developed gardening-in-space program; the plants provide sensory stimulation. The astronauts "love the aromas of the plants," according to Massa. "When they open the door of the plant habitat it's like being in the produce section of a grocery store." Otherwise, the ISS "apparently doesn't smell that great." On a practical level, it's helpful not to have to worry about heaving every bit of food off Earth, hurling it 250 miles up to the International Space Station. Seeds weigh a lot less than full-grown plants, fruits, and vegetables. But space gardening programs are also being developed as a psychological balm for astronauts who might spend up to a year locked in tight quarters with a few other people, cooped up except for occasional turns bouncing around in space.

The program highlights our powerful human need to connect with our food. Back here on Earth, research shows that growing food may have disease-preventing powers. Also known as ecotherapy, horticultural therapy, or agrotherapy, gardening has received attention lately as a new way to provide physical activity, purpose, fresh food, and therapeutic benefits. Research shows that nature-assisted therapy reduces stress and blood pressure, improves cognitive function, and can promote cooperative behavior. There are lots of theories about why gardening has such a profound impact. Gardening decreases the stress hormone cortisol. Also, some evidence shows that dirt has beneficial microbes that can enter the bloodstream when you touch the earth, then enter the nervous system.

It's easier to go to the grocery store than cultivate a green thumb, so many of us have given up on the positive influence that growing food— even just a potted herb sprig on your windowsill—can provide. As modern humans become increasingly removed from the production and preparation of meals, some go to extremes to satisfy our craving for connection to our food. The irony is not lost on me: 200 years ago my ancestors subsistence-farmed so I could live a better life, and now I'm paying to send my kid to a week of farm camp to pick lettuce under the hot sun.

You can buy backyard chickens for fresh eggs or, if you're just chicken curious, you can rent them. In Washington, DC, there are businesses that specialize in loaning chickens to urban dwellers. Or you can rent to own and buy when your lease is up. Williams Sonoma offered a $2,000 chicken coop, and Neiman Marcus once had a $100,000 "Beau Coup," a coop modeled after Versailles. (Included: three heritage chickens and a "library with books"; no word on whether the chickens arrive knowing how to read or if you need to teach them.) The advertising text reads, "You've always fancied yourself a farmer—now . . . you're doing it the fanciest way possible!" Beaucoup, by the way, is French for "a lot." Indeed.

For some perspective on our need to connect with agriculture, let's look back a century or so. Until advancements in transportation like refrigerated trucks eliminated spoilage concerns, fresh food mostly came from farms around one's home. The average grocery store we recognize today is a modern miracle, an Eden down the street, with fresh food from every corner of the globe and enough shelf-stable food to keep a person alive for her natural life. (Of course, that natural life span might be short-ened by some of the food we find in an average grocery store.)

One of my ancestors was an indentured servant who came over on the *Mayflower*, and I often wonder what he and his crewmates, many of whom starved to death through the first winter, would have done if they walked into a grocery store. Collapse to their knees? Weep? Just look at a grocery store's cheese section—not even the fancy cheese, just the wall of cheese in the dairy aisle. How many ways can you buy cheddar cheese in a grocery store? The last time I was in one I counted, and it's at least 28—I may have missed some.

For most of the modern grocery store's history (about 100 years since the first Piggly Wiggly), the stores haven't had windows. Sure, there may be large windows at the front, but few or none actually in the store. This is part of general retail psychology, to turn stores into places of fantasy; the goal is to transport you to a time and place removed from the outside world so you buy more. There are no health consequences to processed foods when you can't even see a world outside the grocery store.

Companies are now creating entire housing developments centered on farming. Known as "agrihoods," these communities integrate farms into residential areas and give new meaning to the phrase "mixed-use development."

At one such community in Ashburn, Virginia, homes—which cur-rently sell for between $1 million and $2 million—were developed around a farm conservancy, essentially giving residents access to an enor-mous backyard garden with none of the gardening responsibilities. Devel-opments like this remind me of my son's summer farm experience—good but highly manufactured. The point sometimes isn't so much to create infrastructure to make the community self-sustaining; it's to acquaint non-farmers with agriculture, to scratch the 10,000-year-old agriculture itch. As a farmer friend assured me as I fretted overpaying for farm camp: It's a lot cheaper than owning a farm.

Let's get back to that gardening-in-space program. Astronauts are busy. They already have a lot to do—space exploration, exercise two hours each day just so their muscles don't atrophy in a no-gravity state, draw blood samples and perform other self-experiments, and maintain and repair billions of dollars of equipment. It's not as if space organizations are looking for random fun hobbies, particularly a gardening hobby that requires oxygen, sunlight, and water in a place where none of these exist in abundance. A gardening program was carefully chosen for, among other reasons, its psychological benefits—psychological benefits we see reflected in home chicken coops, agrihoods, and farm camp as ways to spend discretionary income. Being involved with growing your food makes eating a more pleasurable experience, and fresher food tastes better and can have higher nutrient value.

Space is precious in space. Every square inch is accounted for on the International Space Station—no extraneous baggage allowed. Scientists developing space gardens knew the plants must have a low profile, low mass, and use little or no energy. The plants grow on plant "pillows," little packets of a dirt-like growing material (the kind you see on baseball fields and golf courses) and fertilizer pellets that slowly release nutrients that the plants need to grow—nutrients that eventually make their way to the astronauts' bodies when they eat the plants.

Nutrients are important, but astronauts can get them in enriched food created by countries' space food labs. And space food is way better today than the toothpaste-tube beef of the twentieth century: Famed chef Alain Ducasse consults on France's space food program. As French astronaut Thomas Pesquet said, "It's a lot of pressure feeding a Frenchman in space."

"One of the intangibles of having plants in space is having a living piece of Earth with you," Massa told me. When I visited her lab in Cape Canaveral at the Kennedy Space Center, she showed me the growing box, where the plants flourish. The box needed to re-create good growing conditions, including light. When using artificial light, the two colors of light required for plant growth are red and blue. But having only red and blue light in the box would mean that the plants would look an unnatural bright purple to the astronauts; something they would get less pleasure out of growing than a green plant that looked like a plant on Earth.

Purple plants were unacceptable to NASA, as a big part of the program was the research-backed psychological benefit of just looking at plants as they appear on Earth. Bright purple plants would look, well, not like plants. So NASA added green lights to the box for the psychological benefit to the astronauts.

The first lettuces grown on the space station in the mid-2010s had to be propelled back to Earth for studies and to ensure safety—you can barely wash your hands in space, let alone lettuce, and NASA wanted to test for *E. coli* and *Salmonella*. I'm guessing food poisoning on the Space Station is probably even worse than being sick on Earth. Now ISS residents enjoy fresh greens that they use as lettuce wraps and fresh ISS-grown Hatch chiles on their astronaut tacos.

The astronauts breathe the same air as the plants do. They plant the seeds and then thin the seedlings to select only those that have the best chance of growing at the same rate as most other seedlings. They post images of the plants on Instagram. Although there is technology to provide automatic watering, as water forms a ball in space rather than dispersing, the astronauts still sometimes prefer to hand-water the pants. This isn't an easy task. The lack of gravity requires the astronauts to stick their feet under cords to hold themselves down so they stay upright. (Astronauts lose calluses on the bottoms of their feet and develop calluses on the tops when in space for months at a time because of being strapped down rather than pulled down to the ground by gravity.)

The benefits of all these gardening tasks translate to Earth. Astronauts in space are just as excited as we are when we grow something, even though they have the universe at their fingertips. Even with views of the cosmos, they nurture a tiny twig. This is the power of food and the power of growing something.

After ISS astronauts grew the first lettuces in space, which everyone believed to be the first-ever gardening in space, Russian astronaut and Instagram phenom Oleg Artemyev posted a photo of a previously undisclosed sprouting onion. You know when you have an onion on the counter for a while and it starts to sprout a little green sprig? Artemyev brought such an onion on board, unbeknownst to officials, and chopped up the green sprouting part of the onion to sprinkle on his astronaut food. Oleg's onion is a good example of the psychological power of growing something—

of all the things he could sneak on board for a yearlong trip, he chose a sprouting onion. Oleg said that now that they were growing lettuce too, they could make an internationally grown space-salad.

Growing something usually involves touching dirt, which has its own benefits. Leonardo da Vinci wrote: "We know more about the movement of celestial bodies than we know about the soil underfoot." Five hundred years later, it's still true. One teaspoon of healthy soil has more microorganisms than there are humans on earth. And some of them can benefit our gut microbiomes, the constellation of beneficial bacteria that influences our emotional well-being, as we will see in the next chapter.

A 2004 study at the University of Texas found that the nutrient value of 43 crops has decreased since 1950, they believe in part because of less healthy soil from less biodiversity (fewer types of plants grown in an area). According to this research, your food is literally less nutritious now than when your grandmother ate the same meal. This is one reason that it's possible to be both overweight and malnourished. Studies show that higher nutrient levels affect food's organoleptic qualities—taste, aroma, and mouthfeel—and how the human senses detect a food's unique flavor. So less nutritious food may be less pleasurable food.

In addition to soil's benefit of helpful microbes, some research shows the sense of accomplishment that comes with growing your own food prevents depression and antisocial behavior. Sander van der Linden, professor at Princeton University, studies green prison programs, and his research supports that gardening is linked to improved prisoner behavior and less violent prisons. "Even when using the most conservative estimates I could find, I still found large and significant differences—there is definitely something unique about green prison programs." The Rikers Island GreenHouse/GreenTeam programs, van der Linden points out, yielded a huge decrease in prisoner rearrest rates for those in the gardening program. Rikers is one of the most violent correctional complexes in America.

Most of us would agree that creating something makes us feel good. There is a particular satisfaction when you eat food you've grown, and food pleasure can be increased when you are involved, in any way, in thoughtfully procuring it. Growing fresh herbs on your windowsill offers psychological need satisfaction (a scientific way to say happiness) and results in a plant with nutrients. All you need is a pot and a window. (Or not—there are now several companies that sell beautiful, if a little pricey, indoor gardens with LED lights that allow you to grow food anywhere in your home.)

The satisfaction that comes with connecting with how your food is grown can come in other ways too; you'll find some recommendations in Chapter 6.

Cooking and Eating

Our brains find out what is happening around us through the nervous system processing sensory information—what we smell, taste, see, hear, and touch. As we have seen, the nervous system regulates, processes, or controls much of what makes us who we are: consciousness, thought, learning, memory, voluntary and involuntary behaviors, emotion, and sensory perception.

The nervous system is an ancient system. As with emotions, it gives our bodies the ability to turn external stimuli like odors and sounds into electrical and chemical activity that our bodies and brains can process and react to—events/sights/sounds go in, thoughts/feelings/actions come out. The sound of sizzling food causes vibrations in the air. The information of that sound is transmitted throughout the body by neurons throughout the nervous system. We act according to how we process the sound—are we actively cooking or does the sizzle remind us that an empty pan was inadvertently left on the hot stove?

No one quite understands why each brain interprets individual experiences differently, but we believe that how your neurons carry electrical and chemical messages has something to do with it. The brain wants to make sense of things; as researcher and academic Brené Brown has written, "We are a meaning-making species." Your neurons want to process, explain, and give meaning to experiences they're carrying messages about.

And the nervous system relies in part on the experiences you've had in the past and in part on sensory quirks that we aren't aware of.

For all we think about food as sustenance, work, and pleasure, unconscious activity happens with our sensory information while we're eating. Charles Spence researches how senses influence flavor. "It doesn't feel as if my blue coffee cup makes my coffee taste worse," says Spence, even though he has specific research that coffee tastes best in a white cup. "We all believe we can taste just on our tongues, even though the research all says differently." If we know about our sensory eccentricities, we can use them to support short- and long-term emotional wellness through food.

And then there is the curveball of neuroplasticity, that the brain changes without us knowing about it. If you started learning to play piano tomorrow, your neurons may change the way they communicate, and maybe even their structures, so you can create a new skill. Same with cooking. But this neuroplasticity works both ways—if you don't use particular neurons, they may die or thin their portfolio of things they're capable of doing so they can connect with only a fraction of other neurons they used to connect with.

Cooking is not always fun. It is not always relaxing. It is not always a creative outlet. But research shows it's very important to make the effort. When we use our senses more fully, cooking or preparing food can enhance our enjoyment of it and keep those neuron paths going—even when we're just trying to put supper on the table.

Our nervous systems can be calmed by paying attention to our senses, a method referred to as "mindfulness." Observing your senses as you're eating and cooking is an act of mindfulness, and there is lots of research showing that mindfulness is beneficial for emotional wellness and regulation.

There are even therapists who offer mindful cooking classes, otherwise known as "breaditation."

Cooking has historically required significant time: finding foods, harvesting and cooking hard grains, baking bread over fires, hunting and taking apart animals. It was the foundation of what humans did every day. Eating well no longer requires lots of time or any prep at all. We need motivation for when we're peering into the pantry and considering another night of take-out.

"Why cook?" is a real question, not just for people who don't cook but for those of us who have to do it all over again every single day. The dinner fatigue is real. There are a million ways to live in this world that don't involve cooking and can still serve your physical health. But using food to support mental health is more complicated than just choosing the right nutrients because of food's deep connection to how we perceive the world.

Researchers have studied "psychological need satisfaction," also known as the joy of making things. Known in psychology as the IKEA effect, it's the idea that people put more value on something they had a part in creating. As researchers at Harvard Business School put it, "labor leads to love."

Our obsession with food television and food competitions, starting about 25 years ago, has been either the partial cause or the partial result of us not cooking. There are lots more people watching chefs on TV, but the number of people who actually cook has decreased (the same has happened for the number of people who watch pornography versus number of people actually having sex). We'd rather watch the slickly produced facsimile of real life than embrace our own messy reality.

When I was on a cooking competition show for a few months, Chef Bobby Flay wisely said that getting people to actually cook your recipes is the holy grail. I took this to mean that a lot, maybe most, food content is used by people for entertainment purposes only. I'm not demonizing looking at slick photos of food and drizzling caramel in videos and people eating and laughing together on television. Where it starts not to serve us is when we substitute that content consumption for the sensory experience of actual joyful eating or cooking, when we confuse the satisfaction we get from watching and looking with the actual psychological need satisfaction that all humans crave.

The pleasure we've squeezed out of the onslaught of food television for the past two and a half decades of watching people make things and then eat them is transferred need satisfaction. We gather around the glow of a screen like the glow of a fire our ancestors ate around, hearing stories of where the food came from, when what we really want is a glowing hearth in our own homes.

Food television at times sets up unreasonable expectations rather than being aspirational in a positive way, encouraging us to do this at home. When I was trying to explain pornography to my son, I said it's like watching a hockey movie versus playing a hockey game. When you play, there's the time preparing in the locker room, there are conversations behind the plays, there's practice, there's passing back and forth, there are shots on goal that don't make it in. But when you see a hockey movie, it's all action and close-ups of ice spraying everywhere and goal after goal after goal. Entertainment and real life are just different, but entertainment can set our (unrealistic) expectations. And expectations can ruin three fundamentals of life: cooking, sex, and parenthood.

Cooking can be a love language. Like all acts of love, it doesn't have to be complicated. We get so entranced by watching perfect experiences, we can't see the reality in front of our faces. One big rule in food television is that the viewer must always see someone eating. It's not enough to show a finished product. You need the voyeuristic and vicarious pleasure of watching someone enjoy what was made.

Food preparation can be a powerful act of self-care. We extol the virtue of showing love to others through food. How about showing some love to ourselves?

Small acts of creativity every day are crucial to mental health. Cooking counts, even if the results aren't Insta-worthy. I like pictures of a seven-layer sandwich or a perfectly coordinated lunchbox as much as the next person. I once spent minutes mesmerized by a photo of a glass-door refrigerator that was arranged by color. I used to review restaurants where the check came in a hollow, mouth-blown, decorated egg—gorgeous and smashed open in front of you so your bill could escape it. But striving to live that photo-perfect life with every meal you eat is exhausting.

And preparing food is a distinctly sensorial experience involving our nervous systems. Every minute of cooking, our minds use our senses to create perceptions that affect how we enjoy our meals. There is a whole field of science, called neurogastronomy, dedicated to how the brain perceives food, focusing on our emotional, cognitive, and rational enjoyment of what we eat. It's mind hacking for food lovers.

This is important because, when it comes to flavor, perception is all we've got, neurogastronomy founder and Yale School of Medicine neuroscientist Gordon Shepherd told me. Shepherd specializes in how our brains create flavor. And it turns out, all our senses are critically important to flavor or how we enjoy food—it's not just the sense of taste.

"There is no flavor in the molecules of food we eat," Shepherd told me. "It's only what our brains perceive to be flavor through the senses." This may seem like scientific splitting of hairs, but it's critical to how our emotions influence our taste for food when the information is processed by our nervous system. What we bring to the table—the brain—is the keystone of flavor.

The power of sensory involvement is taken to extremes in the restaurant industry, as many things have been in the past couple of decades since dining out became a sport, with everyone playing and spectating at the same time. Sublimotion restaurant on Ibiza, Spain, was designed by engineers, illusionists, set designers, architects, choreographers, and screenwriters who create dining settings like glaciers or volcanoes, complementing them with elaborate costumes and virtual reality (complete with VR glasses). The surroundings change with each course to accompany each unique dish. A survey of Michelin-starred restaurants ranked Sublimotion as the most expensive in the world; prices start at $2,000 per person. At Ultraviolet restaurant in Shanghai, each course is paired with 360-degree projection of images, scent diffusers, cool-air blowers, and sound. It refers to its 20-course experience as "psycho-taste."

On an everyday level, we can use our senses to gain more food pleasure through preparation. "The preparation of the food, the process of cooking, and also the color, the taste, the smell, are all components of the [sensory] process," says Kuan-Pin Su, the director of Mind-Body Interface Laboratory in Taiwan and the vice dean of China Medical University's medical school in Taiwan.

Preparing food doesn't have to mean doing everything yourself from beginning to end. Food curation is a skill as much as clothing curation.

When someone selects tomatoes and a cheese that pairs well with them and serves them on a beautiful plate with spicy olive oil and crunchy grains of sea salt, some "food people" would say that's not cooking because they didn't have to combine ingredients. (It's not even about the presence of heat or actual "cooking.") The definition of cooking, to me, needs to evolve as we evolved the definition of "family" in the past couple of decades. What makes it cooking? And who gets to decide?

You don't sew your own clothes, but people can still compliment you choosing and putting an outfit together. That is a real, admirable skill (and one that people pay a lot for if you're good at it). To me, "cooking" is the feeling. You feel while you cook, different from feeling while ordering through an app. It's also kind of like exercise in this way. I would much rather read a book than exercise. But I do it because there is something elemental about moving your body, reaffirming that you're alive. Sometimes you're happy with the result. Sometimes not. But there is purpose in the process.

SMELL AND TASTE

The oldest model for inducing depression symptoms in animals is removing the olfactory bulb; that's how important smell is for emotional well-being. When mice can't smell, the changes in brain chemistry and behavior look very much like human depression. Further, loss of smell in humans is often followed by depression, as people feel isolated from smells of all familiar things that alert their minds that comfort is nearby.

Olfactory loss changes parts of the brain that regulate metabolism, social behavior, and sexuality. How the olfactory system affects metabolism, and how metabolism affects the olfactory system, is a new area of research—we know there are insulin receptors in our olfactory bulbs, and that is one of the reasons why we are more sensitive to food odors when we are hungry. (Insulin helps the body convert the energy of food into energy in our cells.)

One researcher told me the story of a chef who had a head injury and completely lost the sense of smell. The only thing the chef could eat was Cinnabon. This was interesting because I associate Cinnabon so strongly with the smell that hits you from hundreds of feet away in shopping malls. I have never been surprised by a Cinnabon. Cinnabon announces itself. But the chef loved it, in part, because of the sensation of extreme sweetness. When smell wasn't a part of eating, experiencing sweetness and the chewy texture were the pleasures the chef craved.

People who don't experience smell (called anosmia, for smell blindness) still experience taste—sweet, salty, sour, bitter, umami—but not flavor. Taste comes from our about 10,000 taste receptors on the tongue. Taste thresholds are modulated by neurotransmitters like serotonin and noradrenaline, which are also neurotransmitters related to mental health. "General anxiety level is directly related to taste perception," as one study states.

That's why head injuries can result in both loss of smell and complete loss of flavor memory (the ability to recognize and identify something you've eaten before). "This is puzzling even to a scientist," Yale neurogastronomy researcher Shepherd says. But it shows one thing clearly: We know something complicated is going on in the brain when we savor food. Shepherd asserts that, when you look at the many mechanisms involved in creating flavor, it "engages more of the brain than any other activity or behavior."

That's because the brain uses smell to create flavor. Here's a practical experiment to show what this means. Pinch your nose and bite into a jelly bean, something that would usually burst with flavor when you bite into it. But if you're holding your nose, you won't taste a distinguishable flavor, just sweet. Your brain doesn't create the specific flavor (grape or cherry or orange) because it uses smell to create flavor, and you're pinching your nose. Once you let go, the flavor will come rushing in because you can smell again and the brain now has the tools it needs to create the flavor. And, curiously, the brain creates flavor only when it breathes out, not in. This is surprising because, when we sniff in, we smell all kinds of things in the world—flowers, gas fumes, smoke. But flavor is created in the opposite way, only when we breathe out.

Flavor is created through a partnership between the nose and your brain. Odors are molecules. The nostril has about 360 odor receptors, and there are a trillion distinct odors, so some receptors can be activated by more than one odor. It's as if the receptors have a lock on them, and the lock can be opened with several different kinds of keys. Something we smell—say, chocolate—can have hundreds of different molecules that create it, and the molecules might unlock dozens of different odor receptors.

The receptors send odor information to the brain, and the brain tells you what odor it is and how you feel about it. This process is so integrated with flavor that most people can't separate smell and taste unless they are specially trained for it, usually in the flavor or perfume industries. Training can be months or years long, consisting of smelling different odors to retrain the brain to recognize and identify subtleties.

Smell is a peculiar sense, as it's the only one that isn't regulated by a brain region called the hypothalamus that, as covered in the last chapter, is part of the limbic system (your thumb in the hand model of the brain) and sends information to other parts of the brain. Sight, sound, touch, and taste all go through the hypothalamus, but smell doesn't work that way. Smell has its own special area, an ancient part called the olfactory cortex. Receptors in the nose connect to the olfactory bulb, which then connects directly to the other parts of the limbic system—the amygdala (the almond, the emotional center of the brain) and the hippocampus (the seahorse, the center of memory). There is no mediation between the olfactory bulb and the very ancient and very emotional amygdala, so your sense of smell engages the brain in ways that the other senses do not.

You may recall that the amygdala regulates perception of threats. This may be why smell is so closely related to emotional memories and some smells are wonderful to people, while others find them repulsive. In one study, showing participants photos along with releasing an odor resulted in people using more emotionally charged words to describe the photo than those who experienced no odor when seeing the photos. Smell adds dimension to our lives. Even as our brains grow and change and new cells are made, smell memory remains.

In this way, smell works through your unconscious mind. And it's why some people's immediate reactions to smells are so personal. If you have a bad memory attached to a smell of, say, a certain deodorant or shampoo, you probably don't like that scent. And you may react poorly to someone who uses the same soap because they smell like someone who hurt you years ago.

To test the human sense of smell—which we know is less sensitive than some animals' sense of smell, including dogs—researchers recruited 32 students at the University of California, Berkeley for a study that was later published in the journal *Nature Neuroscience*. The students met in the campus quad and were blindfolded and equipped with thick gloves, kneepads, elbow pads, and earmuffs. They were asked to crawl on the grass and try to track the scent of chocolate from one point to another. The chocolate scent, unknown to the participants, was sprayed onto a 30-foot piece of twine that snaked through the quad. (They couldn't feel the twine because of the gloves and padding, and couldn't hear where other students were because of the earmuffs.) The majority of participants could follow the scent trail with no input from any of their senses other than smell.

We have an unconscious bias to sniff out things that will give us the most sustenance, left over from a time when we had to forage for food. It is likely that odors give some indication of nutrient content, which may be one reason that smelling high-calorie foods makes you want those high-calorie foods. (We have taste receptors for fat that indicate "fat" to the brain when we taste a fatty food, so the idea of odor receptors for fat is not so far-fetched.)

Our sense of smell identifies whether a food has a lot of fat or just a little; it can lead us to seek out high-fat foods as the energy-hungry hunters and gatherers we still are biologically. Sensory perception is based on more than just our physical reality. Sense perception is a feedback loop that happens in your brain between odors and food intake. At Northwestern University School of Medicine, one lab showed that different states of mind affect how sensitive we are to odors. In one 2021 study, participants fasted for six hours and then were exposed to an odor that was a combination of food and nonfood (for example, pizza and pine). When hungry, they perceived the food odor as the dominant odor—even when the percentage of food odor was much lower than the nonfood odor. When participants had just eaten, however, they didn't identify the food odor as dominant as much. A hungry subject, for instance, would smell in a 50/50 mixture of cinnamon bun and cedar odors but identify cinnamon bun as the dominant odor. If that person had just eaten cinnamon buns, the cinnamon bun odor had to increase to 80 percent before being identified as dominant. MRI scans of participants' brains confirmed that the odor-processing parts of the brain were different when participants were hungry versus when they were full.

This matters, as many studies show that we eat what we smell. People who were exposed to a pear odor, for example, were more likely to choose a fruit dessert over a chocolate dessert.

"Our sense of smell is as individual as our fingerprints," smell researcher Dr. Nancy Rawson explains. "We all live in a different sensory world when it comes to aroma. We all live in different olfactory worlds."

The memory of smell remains even though the ability to smell declines significantly as we age. Because of the direct connection of smell to emotional memory, it allows our minds to travel back in time to places and emotions that we associate with odors.

When we smell something that we smelled when we were comfortable, confident, cared for, we will have less of a stress response. The brain gets into association patterns. For me, it's the smell of boxwood, a bush that my grandmother had in her garden in Queens when I was very young. Her home was something of a sanctuary, as I could walk there alone and just sit with her in her garden. And smelling boxwoods always brings me back to that, so I have several in my own front yard now. Whenever I walk by them, I travel back in time to that safe space in the middle of chaos.

Smell as time-travel or place-travel or emotion-travel is particularly apparent in elderly populations. The sense of smell is critical for maintaining food enjoyment in the elderly, who often experience decreased sense of smell that goes with aging and subsequent decreased quality of life.

We know you can sell your home more easily if something is baking, like bread or cookies—this is because warmer temperatures make the odor molecules more volatile and can produce a stronger, more intense effect in humans. Why not make your home smell comforting all the time by cooking something? We can create that pleasure and anticipation by doing even a small step of food preparation in our own homes.

SIGHT, SOUND, AND TOUCH

In January 2022 the Italian Cultural Centre in Vancouver had a brilliant idea about using food to calm people. Their usual programming included book clubs on great Italian authors, mozzarella classes, a capocollo (known to many Italian Americans as "gabagool") workshop, and pasta-making lessons. But they also started providing Covid-19 vaccinations and requiring people to wait for 15 minutes—often anxiously—to see if they had any adverse physical reactions to vaccination. Most vaccination clinics offered a little space for people to sit and stare into space or scroll on their phones. But at this clinic in Vancouver, Italians were running the show. So, after people received shots, the Italian Cultural Center showed food videos.

I am half Italian American; my grandfather's last name (and my last name for the first 30 years) was Zupa, which means "soup," and my grandmother's last name was Dolce, which means "sweet." So in my experience, the association around the world between Italy and food is a stereotype, but it's also not wrong. Italians are known for using both passionate emotions and great food to live la dolce vita (the good life), no matter what is happening in the world.

At the clinic, patients watched videos of someone stirring an enormous steaming vat of tomato sauce, tiny pools of olive oil gathering on the surface and then being incorporated back, again and again, into a swirl of red gravy. Videos of layering lasagna—handmade noodles, meat, cheese. You can almost taste the acidic-sweet tomato bite of thick sauce in the back of your mouth, feeling a little burn on the tip of your tongue because you didn't wait long enough for the sauce to cool. Watching food being made carefully and lovingly is a calming experience.

You may have heard the phrase "we eat first with our eyes," attributed to the first-century Roman Apicus, who loved food and luxury. (Same, Apicus.) Researcher Charles Spence—the one who looks at why coffee has worse flavor in a blue cup than in a white cup—has made a career showing that Apicus's saying is true and examining the effects of sound and touch too. Spence is a winner of the Ig Nobel Prize, which is awarded to unusual research that "at first makes people laugh, and then makes them think." He is the best combination of curious, nutty, and smart. When he was just 28 years old, he was offered his own research lab at Oxford. The last time we spoke before we talked recently was years ago, when I was researching flavor creation for *National Geographic*. He hasn't changed.

When I interviewed him by video recently, he was in Colombia during the rainy season and his internet connection kept going out, but every time I could see there was a taxidermied goat head on his wall, with a top hat, smoking a cigar. When I asked him about it, he said, "You know, Churchill." I guessed this was in reference to the top hat and cigar Churchill often donned, but with a shaky internet connection I couldn't waste time chatting about that. After we talked, I did some cursory googling about it for a while, but all I found were articles about how they use goats to calm down the horses at Churchill Downs before the Kentucky Derby. I still don't know what the goat head means, other than an unflattering comparison of Churchill to a goat. But you get the idea of who Spence is.

Spence is the clinical godfather of using the senses to heighten food experiences. He consults with high-end restaurants on using his research to enhance dining and ensure a chef's food puts its best foot forward. Spence's research makes you question everything you thought you knew about flavor because he shows that senses other than taste affect how you enjoy food, perhaps even more than taste.

Spence's research found that food tastes sweeter when served on a white plate than on a black one. Changing from rectangular slate plates to round white ceramic plates made the same dessert taste a further 10 percent sweeter.

The color of food is also critically important. According to Spence, "Color is the single most product-intrinsic sensory cue when it comes to setting people's expectations regarding the likely taste and flavor of food and drink." (Anyone who has ever had a child ask for "red flavor" juice can attest to this.) Foods that are colored more intensely, even by dyes, are identified as more intensely flavored.

Spence has conducted similar experiments with wine. In one study, professional sommeliers believed that they were drinking red wine when their glasses were actually full of white wine with red food coloring. (People love to fool professional sommeliers.) At the University of Bordeaux, fifty-four participants were asked to smell and describe two wines, one red and one white. Participants gave vastly different descriptions of the two wines they smelled. The catch: They were the same white wine, but one had food coloring in it. The resulting paper was titled, "The Color of Odors."

Spence ran a study at a retirement home for British actors, entertainers, and circus professionals, Denville Hall. (Denville Hall could be its own book.) He and a chef wanted to see if multisensory nostalgia could increase elderly residents' enjoyment levels of nutritious food. They served easy-to-eat savory ice creams made from nutrient-rich familiar tastes from their childhoods—tomato soup and shrimp salad were two. At the same time, they projected photos and played music from participants' younger years. As Spence suspected, nostalgic sights and sounds and flavors boosted participants' enjoyment of their food. In psychology there is a theory that all memories from adolescence and our early twenties are particularly emotionally powerful. This power is known as the "reminiscence bump," and it was on full display at Denville Hall.

Food is further perceived as fresher and tasting better when it has visible fresh herbs, regardless of the flavor the herbs provide. Because flavor is created in your brain, your food will have better flavor with the herbs even if your food doesn't have better taste with the herbs. So, when you have a recipe that tells you to finish by sprinkling some fresh herbs on top of the finished dish, sometimes you're standing in the grocery store like, *do I really need these? I'm going to use only a few leaves. All I need is a teaspoon, and now I have to buy this enormous bunch of chives.* Yes, you need them if you want food with better flavor.

Sound can be a secret ingredient for pleasurable eating. "Sonic seasoning" describes how sound affects flavor in the brain and our enjoyment of food. What we hear can make food taste sweeter or lighter or more bitter. In

Spence's Ig Nobel–winning study, known as the "sonic chip" experiment, he showed that we eat with our ears in addition to the other senses. Subjects were seated in a sound booth and ate potato chips of varying degrees of freshness—some chips were right out of the package, some were stale. Spence and his colleagues intermittently piped crunching sounds into the booth. People who ate the stale chips with no sound thought the chips were pretty gross, as expected. But people who ate stale chips and heard crunching noises rated the chips as 15 percent crunchier than when they ate the same stale chips with no crunching noise. Sound worked on the brain to increase perceived freshness and crunchiness of the chips.

Other examples: Drinking whiskey in a bright room while listening to the sounds of a lawnmower and birds will make your drink taste grassier; drink it while listening to a fire burning, and it will taste woody. When bacon-and-egg ice cream was served with sounds of sizzling, it was rated as tasting more like bacon. When it was served with sounds of chickens clucking, it tasted more like eggs. Everything matters in the dining experience, and chefs, who make their living off perceived deliciousness, know this is true.

If you are a person who follows restaurant trends, you may remember "Sound of the Sea." The title refers to a dish that the British restaurant The Fat Duck introduced in 2007, a seafood dish on a bed of edible "sand" and "shells" that came with an iPod playing ocean sounds recorded directly from the English seaside. The food on the plate was razor clams, sea urchin, oysters, and seafood foam, with "sand" made from tapioca and panko bread crumbs. The dish's effect was so much more than what was on the plate. People cried when they ate it, recalling memories of childhood, deceased relatives, happy times gone by. Sound of the Sea and its creator, Chef Heston Blumenthal, became an international restaurant phenomenon. (Spence consulted on its creation.)

We know that music generally can quickly change our emotional state, so why not our food perception? It's not surprising that fast music increases eating speed and slow music decreases it. But slow music also increases perceived food quality. Also, according to a chef research pair's study, "lower-pitched vibrational bass sound made the dessert [toffee] more bitter and brought out burnt notes, while a high-pitched sound made the toffee more sweet and floral."

Touch is critically important in appreciating food. Touch generally informs all the senses. The molecules that make up odors touch your smell receptors for smell, light touches your eyes to produce sight. In the book *Touch: Recovering Our Most Vital Sense*, Richard Kearney argues that touch is a double sense in this way.

Mouthfeel is a branch of touch. Some researchers consider the tongue as a "measuring instrument" that can determine whether we like a food. My toddler son loved broccoli stalks but hated the tops because of the way they felt in his mouth. When he was very little, he would take an experimental bite of the top and spit it out, wipe off his tongue, then hungrily and happily eat the bottoms.

Mouthfeel can be affected by so many things, as Cadbury found out years ago. Cadbury's Dairy Milk bar in Britain is a mouth-coating milk chocolate experience, so beloved that some Brits ship bars to friends in America (full disclosure: I have been one of those American friends). One of the main differences between the British and the American Cadbury bar is that there is higher milk fat in the British chocolate, giving more mouth-coating meltiness. Another difference is that in Britain, fats such as palm oil and shea butter may be used in milk chocolate; in the United States, the law doesn't allow them to be used. So the mouthfeel is different.

In the early 2010s, Cadbury changed its chocolate bars from rectangular pieces to round pieces. According to research, people associate round foods with sweetness and rectangular foods with bitterness. So, although the formula for the chocolate hadn't changed, the perceived taste was sweeter.

Dairy Milk was a long-beloved UK product, introduced in 1905, and Cadbury swears its Dairy Milk chocolate recipe has not changed. According to Spence, who later wrote on the phenomenon of the round chocolate bar, chocolate eaters were "writing and phoning-in in droves (though exact numbers are understandably hard to come by) to voice their concern about what has happened to their much-loved Dairy Milk bar. In particular, many of them have been complaining that the new, rounder format bar tastes 'too sweet.'"

Spence argued years ago that it could have been an opportunity for Cadbury—they could have changed the shape and quietly reduced the sugar in the recipe at the same time, keeping both consumers and public health advocates happy.

How you eat can determine what you eat, some studies have shown. Chewers (who eat slowly and less vigorously) or crunchers (who eat more forcefully) use their teeth to break down food (same mouth motions, different intensity), while suckers and smooshers manipulate food between their tongue and the roof of their mouths (suckers tend to suck the flavor out of the food before smooshing).

The process of how you eat is particularly important when it comes to foods like meat substitutes, as the majority of people who don't like "fake meat" claim that texture is a big problem. In a Texas A&M study, researchers found that 45 percent of Americans are chewers, 33 percent are crunchers, 16 percent are smooshers, and 8 percent are suckers. Yes, these are the technical terms. Whether you like meat substitutes—or any other kind of food—depends at least in part on how you break the food down in your mouth. Food researchers for companies know this; most consumers don't. It's one of the countless subconscious preferences that influence what we eat.

Chewers want a burger with a medium moistness—not too dry or greasy. Crunchers want a burger with a crispy exterior, like a smash burger or something from a sizzling hot grill (usually with a higher fat content to make that crunch). Smooshers want a smooth burger with no bits of gristle, and suckers want a burger that is well seasoned before it's cooked. All of this may seem like it's interesting only to industries trying to hock meat substitutes—but it's important to public health and individual health research, too, because it can help us understand why we eat certain things and make decisions in accordance with the science.

"Mouth geometry," as it's called by researchers, influences the way food hits the tongue, how quickly it dissolves, and how flavors are released. This is why when I changed from milk to dark chocolate, it helped to get round dark chocolate pieces—the dark chocolate tasted less bitter to me and dissolved more pleasantly than rectangular pieces. At least it did in my mind—and isn't that the point?

Remember the chef who lost the sense of smell but loved Cinnabon's overwhelming sweet taste? Touch was another sense that influenced enjoyment. The spiciness in cinnamon causes physical rubbing on the tongue, creating a sense of flavor that can enhance, but is separate from, taste.

This tongue irritation is known as chemesthesis. It's what happens when we eat chili peppers too—there is an ingredient in chilis called capsaicin that affects our taste experience based on the capsaicin roughing up our tongues. Chemesthesis can also release endorphins, which is why some people love the feeling of eating something that actually feels painful.

Some people (including me) love sparkling water, in part because carbonation acts like a spice, interacting with nerve endings and taste buds. When the flavor of the water is combined with the physical effects of the bubbles, water becomes more pleasurable to some people. The bubbles and tingling employ the same receptors as cinnamon, mustard, and horseradish. The water doesn't change, but your experience of it—and therefore the amount of pleasure you get out of it—changes based on your particular body and set of experiences. Food can taste sweeter with carbonation and less sweet when cold. The premium carbonated water industry is competitive—everything in the water matters, the size and number of bubbles just as much as the quality of the actual water.

Spence's research further shows that heavy dishes and heavy cutlery create the flavor perception that food is tastier and of higher quality. And for those who crave sodium, food tastes saltiest when sampled from a knife rather than a fork, spoon, or toothpick (although I'm not sure it's worth the risk).

Eating Together

For most of human history, eating alone was not an option. We hunted and gathered and ate in packs to protect ourselves. Now we do the opposite. A 2019 American survey showed that adults eat more than seven meals alone each week. In a 2015 survey, almost 60 percent of Americans often eat alone, and 46 percent of adult meals were eaten alone. And the number of meals eaten alone is increasing.

In another recent survey, half of the people who say they enjoy eating alone say it's because they can relax more. I feel this way a lot too, especially when I get to put drippy natural peanut butter on an apple nugget, sprinkle it with craggy Maldon salt, and pop it into my mouth at the kitchen counter. But I wondered why my brain sometimes finds eating alone more relaxing. And I wondered if I could work with my brain to eat with people more often—a practice that is associated with better health outcomes.

I think of it as the feast paradox: People who eat with others eat more food, but they enjoy better health. Eating with other people may have some protective effect. How is this possible and how can I take advantage of it? As someone who likes eating alone occasionally, how can I use eating as an opportunity to connect with others?

In a world where food is described in moralistic terms ("sinful") and is an indicator of class (McDonald's versus Sweetgreen), eating in public exposes truths about you that may or may not be accurate. Isolating while eating guarantees we won't be judged by other people while we're doing it. If we're alone, we won't be shamed for our choices. We can eat exactly what we want, watching exactly what we want, in whatever manner pleases us. There is a lot of freedom in eating alone, which may be why the incidence of people eating alone increases globally every time a survey is taken. But I also want to work on generally reducing shame around food, which may lead us all to eat more with others and have better health.

Recent science shows that eating with others in today's world can protect us from modern dangers like loneliness, depression, and isolation. And some people report that they have no one to eat with. Thirty-nine percent of Americans say they're not close to anyone, a number that has increased steadily since World War II. A lot of this is due to other changes in society—single-person American households increased from 17 percent in 1970 to 27 percent in 2012.

We often focus on the health benefits of specific foods of the Mediterranean diet without focusing on other cultural aspects of Mediterranean living. The United Nations Educational, Scientific and Cultural Organization (UNESCO) wrote: "Eating together is the foundation of the cultural identity and continuity of communities throughout the Mediterranean basin. It is a moment of social exchange and communication, an affirmation and renewal of family, group, or community identity." It continued, "[Food] markets also play a key role as spaces for cultivating and transmitting the Mediterranean diet."

Rates of loneliness have risen to the point that Surgeon General Vivek Murthy declared loneliness an epidemic in America. While we can't completely equate eating alone and loneliness—we all know you can be in a room full of people and still feel lonely—rates of loneliness have doubled since the 1980s. Loneliness has the same reduction in life span as 15 cigarettes per day.

In a 2013 study, people who believe their lives have meaning have lower genetic expression of inflammation and lower levels of cortisol, both of which can positively influence emotional well-being. If you feel that you have a high purpose in life, your cortisol level comes down more quickly after it's been activated, which can also be a sign of healthy processing of emotions. The amygdala doesn't react as severely to negative stimuli in people who have purpose. Additionally, a meta-analysis of studies with more than 136,000 subjects found that purpose can lower mortality by 17 percent.

Connectedness is so powerful that the Japanese concept of ikigai (life worth living, or sense of purpose) is included in the Japanese Ministry of Health, Labour and Welfare's health promotion. In a study of 43,000 Japanese, subjects had a 60 percent higher risk of dying of cardiovascular disease if they didn't have ikigai. Along the same lines, people with a community around them often have a stronger sense of purpose and meaning.

Food is a tool for connecting, and both cooking and eating with others can create meaning. We know that kids who have family mealtime have a lower incidence of depression, higher grades, and higher self-esteem; adults can benefit too. We need to take care of ourselves and be concerned about our emotional well-being just as we do with children.

People just don't eat with others like we used to, and in isolating, we're losing one of the great opportunities we have to connect with others. When we eat anything, our brains release dopamine, which encourages bonding. The Covid-19 pandemic reminded us all that we often find happiness in the simplest stimuli—a warm bed, a shared meal, a visit with friends. "Entertaining" doesn't have to be a production; it can be as simple as conversation, refreshment, and laughs. Many studies show that people who spend money on experiences, rather than things, are the happiest.

We can find happiness by prioritizing simple pleasures, and good food shared with others can be a shortcut to this happiness. You can create both immediate pleasure and long-term health benefits through sharing a meal, and it doesn't require a drastic change in your routine; you're eating several times a day anyway.

Good food often opens up channels of communication. Brain imaging studies show that verbalizing feelings makes sadness, anger, and fear less intense; the "talking cure" is not only found in a therapist's office. Talking about emotions causes the amygdala, the emotional center of the brain, to become less active, while the prefrontal cortex becomes more active.

And the food doesn't have to be fancy. Journalist Sally Quinn, who has hosted some of the most legendary Washington, DC, dinner parties, once told me she has no problem "entertaining" by serving good food that she picked up at a store (she is partial to Popeyes fried chicken). People are there for the experience of being with other people. She also said if you are not a great cook but you want to cook for people, have exactly one dish that you make really well and tell people on the invitation that they are coming over specifically for that, even if it's simply your spaghetti. "Sally's Spaghetti" is indeed a coveted Washington invitation.

As I've heard it, my great-grandmother cooked for everyone all the time. Her husband, my great-grandfather, owned a bar during Prohibition; he wasn't around much. They emigrated from southern Italy to the Bronx. She didn't own a lot of dishrags—mappina in Italian—so when she needed to wipe her hands, she dragged them down the front of her apron. That is how my father remembers her—cooking in an apron with long hand-streaks of tomato sauce. She "entertained," in our twenty-first-century lingo, cooking for anyone who came over and ate, while covered in tomato sauce.

I love the stories of both Sally and my grandmother because they show the value of being together in two very different worlds and place the experience over the fuss. Having people over to your home and cooking for them is an act of showing who you are, how you exist in the world. That's rare these days. We make lists of things we have to do to prepare for people to come over, buy new linens, move furniture around. Ads for Thanksgiving-specific things arrive in August. It's hard to carefully choreograph every time people gather in your home, so a lot of us just choose not to have anyone over.

As we conflate eating together with performing, and as the rise of food reality television has elevated everyone's view of what food should be, we've distorted eating together to fit it into a narrow box we call "entertaining." Gone is the come-over-for-coffee invitation, replaced by dinner-party expectations. We have grown to expect a restaurant-style experience, both from others and from ourselves.

I'm not expecting cooking shows or cookbooks to show people fighting over politics at the dinner table or shaming someone for heaping food onto a plate. Connections can't happen easily when we're self-conscious at a table, when sharing food is a source of restriction rather than liberation. None of us is Instagram-perfect when we're eating.

Sometimes I want to put a dollop of whole-grain mustard inside a piece of soppressata and eat it like a taco. That combination of pop from the tiny mustard seeds; the unctuous, melty fat of the salami; and the peppery hot flavors is, for 30 seconds, my idea of heaven. Sometimes I spoon the salty nut crumbs from the bottom of a cashew jar and pop them right into my mouth. And even while I write this, I'm concerned that you're judging me. But worrying about food shaming brings some level of social anxiety to every meal with others, which is the opposite of beneficial. So is confusing fantasy with reality, expecting the social media simulacra of our friends and families and famous people to show up to dinner when it's really actual people with histories and feelings and quirks and moles that you can't Photoshop out in real life.

Preparing meals can be a charged subject because, even in the first century, the expectations of home cooking disproportionately affect women. Regardless of gender, after caring for children, being a spouse, holding down a household and/or a job, the idea that we have to impress people in our off-hours is enough to drive us to boxed macaroni and cheese eaten while staring blankly at a screen. When we eat alone, there are no external expectations. But when we eat alone, we lose the connection to others that can enrich our lives, which can feel so depleted by expectations.

In psychology, the term "generous authority" means using your position of authority as a host to protect and serve the group (including yourself). This is one of the best benefits of having people over, and to me, it's always the top goal. Generous authority is concerned with how people connect over a shared purpose, including sharing food (whether spaghetti or a five-course meal). As Priya Parker wrote in her book, *The Art of Gathering*, at some point gathering got tangled up with hosting because the domestic sphere was for a long time one of the only places where women could exert any power. So all the brainpower and intelligence of all the smartest women you know was poured almost exclusively into the domestic sphere. I love the domestic sphere; it's a valuable place to be. But insisting that it was women's only place wasn't good for anyone. Entertaining became mixed up with showing perfection and impressing others rather than the relief of just being your authentic self with friends.

Some of this domestic performance anxiety stems from a change in the reigning dining tradition. About 125 years ago, the prevailing way of serving food went from French service, which is essentially everyone eating off a big platter, to Russian service, which is each individual getting their own plated dinner, with little regard for what specific piece of meat they wanted or how large a portion. This was due in part to the rise of restaurants and the hotel industry, pioneered by the partnership of Chef Auguste Escoffier and hotelier César Ritz. But it also meant that expectations changed from big platters to exquisitely designed individual plates of food.

Because we eat alone so much, a lot of processed-food production is now geared toward solo diners; the market is making products to support doing the thing you want to do but isn't good for you. Single-portion meals in grocery stores have risen every year for the past several decades. But commercials for single-serve meals still often show people eating together.

We blame our 24/7 culture for our bad habits: constant snacking to stay alert, eating lunch at our desks and breakfasts in our cars, dinner grabbed while dashing between commitments. But perhaps our 24/7 culture is both a cause and an effect of us choosing to eat alone more in recent decades. Maybe the trend toward companies marketing snack food was created by our demand and desire to eat alone or on the go, in addition to the other way around. Maybe our own discomfort around owning our food pleasures prevents us from the longer-lasting pleasure of being around people. We eat quickly and lament a world in which things seem cheap and quick rather than satisfying. There's a cognitive dissonance between the kind of eating that we know leads to better emotional wellness and how we actually do eat.

Eating alone as a pattern is a health risk. People who eat most of their meals alone are at increased risk for heart disease. Men who dine alone twice a day are at greater risk for metabolic syndrome, regardless of weight or diet.

In Britain, there is an ongoing national effort called The Big Lunch, encouraging eating together and performing research about the benefits of communal eating, showing that the more often people eat with others, the more likely they are to be happy and satisfied with their lives—to come to that Japanese sense of ikigai. The Big Lunch research, performed with the University of Oxford and published in a paper titled "Breaking Bread: The Functions of Social Eating," shows that communal eating increases well-being, whether it's a feast or a snack. The research looked at the association between eating together and happiness, community connection, and life satisfaction. Responses from the survey showed a strong connection between social eating and social bonding, to the point that "communal eating may have been evolved as a mechanism for humans to do just that."

The mood elevation we get from eating with people is ancient, based in our primal human nature to sit around a fire pit, share food, and tell stories to make sense of our lives. Over millennia, eating together has been imprinted onto our DNA, according to anthropologist Richard Wrangham in his book, *Catching Fire: How Cooking Made Us Human*. There is something distinctly human about the food rituals that spontaneously happen among humans around food. "No one knows how deeply the effects of cooking . . . have been burned into our DNA."

Archaeologist Martin Jones agrees. He wrote in a 2007 study, "The unique ability of the modern human brain brought us to a most unusual behavior pattern, the gathering around a hearth in a conversational circle to share food." People who eat together are more likely to have a ritual before, such as giving thanks. And food rituals can help us eat better. One study mentioned in the introduction showed that having an eating ritual over five days drove participants to choose healthier food. There was some evidence that the increased feeling of discipline that comes with a ritual made for better choices.

Food is a window into our priorities; a commitment to eating with others more often means rearranging priorities—eating together at lunch instead of working more, or taking a break to snack with someone rather than grabbing something in the car. It's about making it a priority to come home in time for dinner. There is nothing more human than sitting down at a table and eating with others while discussing how we feel about the society we've created.

Not to pathologize being alone; I love it and often prefer it. Restaurateur Danny Meyer once told me that people eating alone in his restaurants is the highest compliment they can pay because it shows that the patron loves the place so much, they go there for self-care. A quiet, solitary meal can be a great act of self-care. And sometimes I choose to eat alone *because* it's too complicated (logistically and emotionally) to eat with others.

I'm also not going to tell you every meal with others is a transcendent experience. I'm reminded of the family dinner scene in the film *Little Miss Sunshine* when the mom throws a box of popsicles on the table and shouts, "Dessert!" while nervously biting off a huge chunk of popsicle and gnawing on it. My teeth hurt just thinking about it. As with all relationships in life, it depends on who you're with. For Thanksgiving 2016, the big joke in America was that you couldn't use knives to cut your food at the dinner table because the conversation about politics was so heated. But eating to support emotional well-being is about patterns, not perfection. You don't have to eat every single meal with someone else; try one extra communal meal one week and see how it feels.

There is little research on whether we can get the same effects of eating together with someone on a digital device while on Skype (skeating), Zoom, or FaceTime. Are these any better than the dine-n-scroll that so many of us engage in now? Andy Warhol once said, "I want to start a chain of restaurants for other people who are like me. . . . You get your food and then you take your tray into a booth and watch television." With home and curbside delivery of Michelin-starred meals and streaming media, I think we've effectively achieved Warhol's dream if we want it. But there is a better way to live when long-term emotional wellness is our priority.

Feeding Children

What we feed our kids matters. During a speech at American University, I was asked whether, given limited school funding, I would recommend either feeding kids well or giving them food education. If only we could do both. In 2023, a study of school programs showed that school-based food education, including gardening, cooking, and basic nutrition, both increased the students' unprocessed food consumption and decreased their ultra-processed food consumption. It was the first study to specifically examine the interaction between school-based food education programs and ultra-processed foods.

The purpose of school, of course, is education of all kinds. We teach what we believe to be important and worthy of attention; likewise, what we feed kids in schools normalizes those food choices. In a 2021 survey of school meal programs in 105 countries, high-income students were likelier to receive meals with more fruit and vegetables.

This comes at a particularly critical time of life. A Greek study found that four indicators of mental health are significantly related to breakfast quality and overall dietary patterns in teenagers. The four indicators— self-rated health, body satisfaction, life satisfaction, and mental health symptoms—were significantly better in those who ate a high-quality breakfast, including protein, whole grains, and vegetables.

A study published in 2024 sorted seventy-one adolescents with depression into two groups: one that supplemented the prescription antidepressant Paxil with omega-3 fatty acids (specifically, DHA and EPA) and one that took Paxil alone. The group taking omega-3 fatty acids reported significantly greater improvements in both depression symptoms and cognitive functioning compared with those in the group taking Paxil alone.

Six Ways to Support Your Nervous System with Food

1. **Smell your food.** Breathe in really deeply before you take a bite. Fill your entire belly up and let it expand with the aroma before you fill it with food. Breathing deeply tells your nervous system that it's safe because you can't breathe deeply and slowly when you're physically fighting or running away from something.

2. **Grow a tea garden, big or small, indoors or out.** This sounds like a precious recommendation, but it's easy and a great way to save money on tea. Mint grows like a weed; you almost can't stop it. And a handful of fresh mint leaves and hot water makes a wonderful hot morning drink if caffeine makes you anxious. Working with nature can help the nervous system too. Try growing chamomile.

3. **Move away from the recipe.** Being creative with food can relax the nervous system. Just buying a can of chopped tomatoes, adding herbs and spices as you like them, and letting it simmer for 30 minutes can be a little boost at the end of a long day.

4. **Pick herb leaves.** Fresh herbs usually come on a stem, and picking the leaves off the stem is a small, repetitive activity that requires little brain power but focuses your attention and is satisfying. It smells great too.

5. **ASMR your food.** The autonomous sensory meridian response (ASMR) brings a feeling of well-being and sometimes a tingling sensation. It can be triggered by gentle, repetitive sounds. While some people find listening to food noises annoying, if you're eating alone, try really focusing on the sounds of crunching or slurping or biting.

6. **Keep your blood sugar steady.** Blood sugar can rise for all kinds of reasons, such as physical or emotional stress. High blood sugar resulting from food intake can make the body respond in the same way as it does to stress.

Breaditation Breadsticks

Kneading and rolling little individual pieces of dough gives child-hood Play-Doh vibes that can be the best kind of breaditation—active meditation through cooking.

If making bread seems daunting, either because of your mood or because you've never done it, breadsticks are a perfect choice. You can top them with whatever you feel like—here I've suggested cheese, but you can use sesame seeds or everything bagel seasoning. You can knead some fresh thyme leaves or chopped rosemary into the dough if you feel like it. They're your breadsticks; you get to choose.

MAKES ABOUT 2 DOZEN BREADSTICKS

1 cup warm water

2 teaspoons honey

1 (0.75-ounce) packet active dry yeast

3 cups whole wheat flour

1½ teaspoons kosher salt, plus extra for sprinkling on breadsticks

2 tablespoons extra-virgin olive oil, plus extra for drizzling, greasing, and brushing

¼ cup grated Parmigiano-Reggiano (optional)

In a large bowl, combine the water and honey. Add the yeast and stir with a fork until dissolved. Then add the flour, salt, and 2 tablespoons of the oil and mix with your hands until all the flour is incorporated. Turn the dough onto a floured surface and knead until it is smooth and stretchy (see Note).

Put the dough back in the bowl and drizzle with a little oil. Turn the dough over to coat it with oil. Cover the bowl with a towel and let it sit in a warm corner for about 90 minutes, until the dough is doubled in size. (If you don't know what that looks like, use the camera on your phone to compare.)

Heat oven to 375°F. Line two baking sheets with parchment paper and grease the parchment with oil using your fingers.

Take a sharp knife and cut the dough into equal quarters. Cut each quarter into equal thirds. Roll each piece of dough to about as long as your entire arm and no wider than your pinky (the thinner the dough, the crunchier the breadstick—make sure the width of each piece is about the same). Cut the length of dough into roughly three equal-length pieces and place each on the baking sheet, with a little space in between them so they can puff up. Repeat with the rest of the dough.

Brush the breadsticks with a little oil and bake for about 15 minutes. Remove from the oven, turn with tongs, top with cheese (if using), and bake for another 15 minutes, until both sides are golden brown. Allow the breadsticks to cool if you can stand it and serve alone or with olive oil or marinara sauce for dipping.

NOTE: Don't know what "smooth and stretchy" means? The kneading part is forgiving with breadsticks, so knead for about 5 minutes. Feel how it's different from how it felt when you started kneading? That's how we learn.

CHAPTER 3

The Gut Microbiome

"All disease begins in the gut."
—HIPPOCRATES

"ANYTHING FRAGILE, LIQUID, PERISHABLE, or potentially hazardous?"

I studied the online Postal Service guidelines of what is allowed to go through US mail. In my hand was a plastic envelope with a prepaid label, thin enough that I could just pop it into any standard blue curbside mailbox. The company I purchased it from assured me that would be fine, that they processed all their gut microbiome tests through the US mail. I was uneasy though; the envelope had a tiny vial with my stool sample inside it.

If you had $400 to spend on improving your health, what would you buy? I thought about this a lot when I was looking at purchasing the at-home gut microbiome test that this envelope contained. The companies selling them make all sorts of claims about what knowledge of my gut microbiome could do for me. Personalized food recommendations. Insights into how my health is and where it's going. A group of supplements specifically formulated for me.

The $400 test I held in my hand would, in about six weeks, result in a report with these recommendations. But the diet plan subscriptions, supplements, and other merchandise would carry additional fees.

I bought the test because of the mounting evidence that what happens in the gut microbiome affects emotional well-being. Some findings:

> In one study, volunteers who ate a probiotic—a supplement containing beneficial bacteria—for a month reported less depression; they also had less cortisol in their urine than those who didn't take the probiotic, suggesting that their bodies hadn't made as much cortisol;
> In studies, people with diagnosed anxiety disorders often have an excess of potentially harmful bacteria and vastly different gut microbiomes than people without anxiety disorder; and
> Eating fermented food is associated with lower social anxiety for people with high neuroticism.

The gut microbiome can also influence how your body metabolizes and uses medication, which affects how well the medication works to give the desired effects—and shows that food added to other therapies may be helpful. Some bacteria convert drugs to make them active, and some make them inactive. And some bacteria actually hoard medication so it's not available to your body.

Many more studies are underway, and new gut microbiome discoveries frequently make headlines. I wondered whether knowing more about my own specific situation would empower me. Precision health—knowing exactly what your body is doing at a given moment and being able to address your own personal needs—is a huge industry these days. The past decade alone has seen an explosion in personal-technology health and wellness products to record your steps, your heart rate, your sleep cycles, your blood pressure. And precision medicine research shows a lot of promise to eventually be able to give a patient care that is highly tailored to their personal situation.

I love the idea of opening a report and being told exactly what to do for my specific optimal health. Because every body is different, everybody wants to know about the quirks of theirs. I had already paid the company $400 for the kit and the processing of my sample, so I went to a mailbox and slipped the envelope through the slot. I figured, what's the harm in getting a precision health test done? (Although I know someone who did an at-home DNA test about her ancestry just to find she had a formerly unknown-to-her half-sibling through the test's DNA database. But you can't locate half-siblings through your gut microbiome test, so I decided I was game.)

I wanted to know what all this science means to me specifically. I was excited to identify what bacteria and other microbes are in my gut and learn how I can use that information to better serve my personal health. Company websites have enthusiastic quotes from customers that eating according to their microbiomes gives them more energy and vitality. There were stories about people who tested their microbiomes, were told not to eat a specific food—say, avocados—then lost lots of weight without doing anything else differently. (Maybe they were eating a whole lot of avocados, I don't know.)

I would send my results to some top microbiome researchers I know to see what they thought of the results of my at-home gut microbiome testing. Would the test give me actionable, science-backed personal recommendations?

Before we get to the test results, let's look at why recent compelling gut microbiome research is the science that launched a thousand start-ups. A healthy gut microbiome may be critical for emotional well-being, and food is critical for a healthy gut microbiome.

Gut Microbiome Basics

The "gut microbiome" is the collection of trillions of microbes living in your digestive tract. Most of them live in your large intestine, although the microbes exist in all the hollow organs that food goes through along the digestive system—in your mouth, esophagus, stomach, small intestine, and anus.

Your large intestine is also known as the colon, but probably someone early on wisely decided that people wouldn't get as excited about the "colon microbiome." The large intestine is also sometimes referred to on its own as the "gut." And the large intestine is where most of the microbial action happens. So it can get confusing when people refer to the "gut," and you should always ask exactly what they're talking about. For our purposes, I'll refer to the large intestine as the "large intestine," while the "gut microbiome" will refer to all the microbes along your digestive tract.

Individually, the microbes in our guts are microscopically tiny, but together they weigh an estimated three pounds. Scientists believe that the microorganisms in our digestive tract consist mostly of:

» Bacteria, archaea, and protozoa (three different kinds of microbes that have just one cell);
» Fungi (microbes that can be made up of a single or many cells); and
» Viruses (which reproduce by taking over the host's cells).

People often associate microbes, particularly bacteria and viruses, with bad health consequences. But specific strains and families of microbes—including bacteria and viruses—are highly beneficial for the gut and, research shows, our emotional well-being.

The gut microbiome affects so much of how we experience our daily lives that some scientists call the gut microbiome a "newly discovered organ." (An organ is a bunch of tissues that work together collectively to perform a specialized function, an honorific reserved for things like hearts and brains.) The microbes form communities to work together and perform functions that humans could not perform without them. Microbes predate humans and have coevolved along with us. And each microbe carries its own personal genetic profile—these microbe genes can affect how your human genes behave.

Your human genes carry the information that determines your genetic traits. The human genome describes all of the genes that comprise humans. A gene is found on your chromosomes, which are inside your cells. There can be thousands of genes on one chromosome. It's like a blueprint for making a human. Today's intense study of the gut microbiome is made possible in part by the massive scientific project that mapped the human genome at the turn of the century.

Many of the world's top scientists were surprised by how few genes there are in the human genome, only about 25 percent more than the genome of a fruit fly. Humans have a lot of differences between us, so researchers had hypothesized that individual genetic differences would account for our diversity.

Then we found that humans have 99.9 percent of our genome in common; the blueprint for making me and the blueprint for making Tom Brady or Lil Nas X are only 0.1 percent different. Genes are part of the story about how we experience life, but genes are not the whole story.

TRAUMA AND GENETICS

Around the same time that researchers realized that genetic differences between individual humans are slight, neuroscientists were finding that mice with different gut microbiomes display different levels of anxiety. For instance, John Cryan, the Irish stress neurobiologist who is now deeply involved with nutritional psychiatry, published a study in 2009 showing that animals who have early-life trauma showed differences in their gut microbiomes compared to other animals. Early-trauma animals exhibited more symptoms of psychological problems later in life and also more frequent gut problems, such as irritable bowel syndrome.

By the early 2010s, several studies showed that certain microbes have to be present in animals' guts for their stress responses to work and for their brains to develop properly. Microbial changes affect both the animals' brain chemistry and their behavior.

"The human genome is just one tiny fraction of the genes that are in the human body," gut microbiome researcher Peter Turnbaugh of the University of California, San Francisco, told me. "Microbe cells are fundamentally different than the cells that make up your own tissue."

Many researchers turned from studying genetics to studying variations in microbes living inside of us. If we are all 99.9 percent the same, and if we all have microbes that affect brain function, then perhaps microbes could be part of the explanation of why we are all so different. The National Institutes of Health took note early on. In 2007, a few years after declaring the human genome mapped (although the finality of that claim is debatable), NIH launched the Human Microbiome Project, modeled on the success of the Human Genome Project, to decipher the mysteries of the microbes inside us.

A gut microbiome is like a fingerprint; everyone's is different. The gut microbiome starts being populated the moment you're born—researchers believe that, in the womb, guts are sterile and have no microbes (although they still aren't sure). Babies delivered vaginally pick up microbes from their mothers' birth canals, while babies delivered by cesarean section often have less diverse microbiomes right after birth. There are ongoing studies about how that may affect stress responses later in life (although as someone who delivered my son by C-section, I'm really not looking for more things to feel guilty about). Regardless of our past experiences, can we change our microbiomes now to support emotional well-being?

A healthy person in India and a healthy person in Iceland will have completely different gut microbiomes based on their different foods, environments, and other factors. And your gut microbiome changes a little every day. Some factors that influence your gut microbiome include the microbes specific to where you live, how well you slept last night, whether you exercised yesterday, medication (including but not limited to antibiotics, which kill a lot of the bacteria—both beneficial and harmful—in your gut), age, pets, gardening, your housemates, sex, and your genes. Emotions also influence your gut bacteria—a 2020 meta-analysis showed that "any stressful events experienced by an individual dictates the diversity and composition of their gut [microbiomes]."

Researchers believe there's no one "healthy" microbiome, which is a relief for we who obsess over the perfect diet. That goes for both the total number of microbes and which species of microbes we have inside us. There are about 1,000 possible bacterial species that we know can live inside the gut. During their lives inside your digestive tract, your microbes themselves make substances that affect a lot about the way you experience life, including, potentially, how your human genes express themselves.

In particular, gut bacteria are responsible for making short-chain fatty acids, which protect against inflammation in the body. Chronic inflammation, as we will see in the next chapter, can wreak havoc on our emotional wellness. And chronic inflammation can affect how active our different human genes are.

Most current gut microbiome research focuses on bacteria, mostly because we know how to grow bacteria outside the body, in petri dishes. And in science, you study what you can. It's harder to study a virus, which needs a host to reproduce. (Although researchers have found some bacteria difficult to grow outside the gut because the gut is such a rich and inviting environment for bacteria.) Therefore, a lot of our discussion will focus on bacteria, as does the discussion among most researchers.

This research is exciting for those concerned with food and emotional well-being, and a bit of a relief for those of us who used to fret that our moods might just be in our genes. Genes are unchangeable. But you can change your microbiome. And the thing that changes your microbiome most quickly and consistently is food.

The Gut Microbiome and Emotional Well-Being

Our brain and gut send signals to each other that affect our emotions, mood, and decision-making. This two-way communication system between the gut and the brain is known as the gut-brain loop, or gut-brain axis. The messages they send to each other depend in part on which kind of microbes we have inside us.

A 2019 German study came up with a clever study design to look at how the gut microbiome affects the central nervous system, and production of hormones by the endocrine system. As we know, the nervous system is where we process sensory information into thoughts and feelings. Certain bacteria in the gut microbiome have been shown to suppress stress responses and the production of cortisol. This study wanted to look at ways to "help us improve human behavior, especially in areas such as stress, mood, anxiety, and cognition."

Researchers in Germany used a simple computer ball game to look at how the gut microbiome affects social decision-making. The researchers used a new way to study the brain called magnetoencephalography (MEG). Like fMRIs, MEGs track brain activity. But with MEG you can move around; in fMRIs participants must be perfectly still.

The ability to move around was critical for this particular study. The protocol went like this: During the four-week study, all participants were instructed not to eat any food or supplements containing probiotics or prebiotics and given a detailed list of foods to avoid. Half of the participants were then given a daily supplement containing the bacteria *Bifidobacterium longum*, often found in fermented foods like yogurt, kefir, and sauerkraut. The other half were given a daily placebo supplement. The study was randomized and double-blinded.

Participants also played a videogame called *Cyberball* while having their brains scanned by MEG. *Cyberball* is a simple ball-toss game involving the participant and what the participant believes to be other players. The "other players" are just a computer program, however. You can make the program simulate bullying or prejudice or ostracism by changing variables, such as speed, color, and size of different components of the game.

For the German study, the goal of the game was to make all participants experience social exclusion and rejection. Evolutionarily, social exclusion and rejection were a threat to survival, so our brains are still particularly stress-reactive to these feelings.

The study participant played a three-person ball-tossing game. The participant thought the order of tossing was random. But the other two "people" playing were actually a program designed to exclude the participant. Those two "people" passed the ball back and forth to each other while largely excluding the human participant.

If you've ever been excluded from a game (or anything), you know it can be a stressful experience. Being excluded is everyone's worst playground nightmare. You're back in grammar school and it's recess and your two friends decided they don't want to play with you anymore. It brings back any childhood (or adulthood) memories of being left out, and it's just plain hurtful. Your mind tries to make sense of what is going on and often engages in all kinds of cognitive distortions. These cognitive distortions—they don't like me, there's something wrong with me, I should be embarrassed by being excluded, they're jerks—often have nothing to do with the facts in front of us. Our brains just go to those conclusions because of triggers of being excluded at other times in life or engaging in emotional reasoning. Even thinking about it now makes me feel a little stressed.

All participants showed some brain changes that indicated the kind of stress response that the game was designed to induce. But during the game there was less stress activity in the brain in participants who had taken *Bifidobacterium longum*. Additionally, those participants' resting stress level was lower, which, researchers wrote, "may be involved in the counter-regulation of negative emotions." The game was the same for everyone, but the *Bifidobacterium longum* had an effect on decreasing or eliminating people's negative responses to the ball being kept away from them. It took a potentially negative emotional experience and made it neutral.

In 2021, John Cryan's lab released results of a study that essentially took Felice Jacka's SMILES trial—the first randomized trial showing that food and mood were associated, back in 2011—and bolstered the Mediterranean diet by adding more fiber and fermented foods, which our good gut microbes thrive on. The trial followed 50 stressed people with formerly poor nutrition for one month. Symptoms of anxiety, stress, and depression went way down after the subjects followed the microbiome-enhancing diet. According to Cryan, "The social brain is very sensitive to changes in the microbiome."

It's easier, given current ethical standards adopted by the science community, for scientists to track constant brain activity of animals than that of humans. Some significant animal research includes findings like:

» When the microbiomes of anxious humans were transferred into healthy mice, the mice subsequently exhibited stress behaviors, such as giving up more easily in a swim test.

» In one study, when mice were fed the beneficial bacteria *Lactobacillus*, their brains showed an increased number of cells that were receptive to GABA, a neurotransmitter that regulates anxiety.

» In a study of 416 human twin pairs in Britain, a certain family of bacteria was more common in individuals with lower body weight than in obese individuals. When those specific bacteria were transplanted into mice, the mice gained less weight than untreated mice.

» A 2022 study in mice showed that the gut microbiome can influence brain plasticity, including adapting better to change.

» When rats exhibiting depression symptoms ate the probiotic *Lactobacillus* (found in yogurt), the depression symptoms reversed.

» Transferring the microbiome of obese people into healthy-weight mice tends to make the mice obese too.

» Transferring the microbiome of people with schizophrenia leads healthy mice to exhibit symptoms of schizophrenia.

» Microbes in fruit flies' guts influenced the insects' food choices. Fruit flies with particular bacterial species in their microbiomes ate more protein. When researchers changed the flies' microbiomes, the flies ate more sugar.

Mice without a microbiome, so-called "germ-free mice," had different brain structures and behaved significantly differently than mice with typical microbiomes. Also, brain disorders progressed far more rapidly in germ-free mice. Some microbes made symptoms of ALS (Lou Gehrig's disease) better, some microbes made symptoms worse. And the amygdalae (the emotional center of the brain) of germ-free mice perform differently than the mice with gut microbes, potentially compensating for the lack of mood-regulating gut bacteria.

In studies, the microbiomes of healthy mice were transplanted into stressed mice. The stressed mice then showed fewer anxiety symptoms. And when the microbiomes of stressed mice were transplanted into healthy mice, the healthy mice showed more anxiety symptoms, for example, avoiding certain parts of a maze. When mice exhibiting depression symptoms were given a healthy microbiome transplant, their inflammatory profile decreased too.

One experiment I referred to in the first chapter tested the effectiveness of the antidepressant/anti-anxiety medication escitalopram (Lexapro) versus beneficial bacteria supplements in stressed mice. In a research lab, scientists may induce stress in mice by giving them a confounding task, such as putting them in a maze. And effects of stress can be measured by giving the mice an endurance task, such as the swim test, after the maze to see how well they do. Stressed mice were given escitalopram, or one of two bacteria heavily studied for alleviating depression and anxiety symptoms, or nothing. Then the mice had a stress test. Both varieties of bifidobacterium and the escitalopram made the mice perform equally well in some stress tests.

Gut bacteria also help make brain chemicals we need for mental health, neurotransmitters that regulate mood and emotion, such as dopamine and serotonin. About half of the body's dopamine is made in the gut, which is also where up to 90 to 95 percent of serotonin is manufactured. Certain gut flora encourages production of serotonin and other neurotransmitters. Serotonin deficiency can be caused by not eating enough of the food that is needed to make serotonin, such as tryptophan or vitamin B_6.

The gut microbiome regulates a lot of body functions that affect emotional wellness—influencing digestion and metabolism, extracting calories and nutrients from your food, regulating your body's immune system, and killing bad bacteria.

How the Brain and Gut Connect

We don't—and likely never will—understand the brain entirely. But we do know some nervous-system mechanisms through which the gut and brain communicate. Two major areas of research are the enteric nervous system and the vagus nerve. They are both parts of the autonomic nervous system, which we'll discuss next.

THE ENTERIC NERVOUS SYSTEM

Your digestive system has its very own nervous system, and it's talking to your brain. And what is in your gut microbiome can influence what it says.

Let's take a quick review of the nervous system, the body's high-speed communication system. Think of a tree dividing into two trunks at its base. The central nervous system (CNS), which consists of the brain and spinal cord, is one trunk. The other trunk is the peripheral nervous system (PNS), which is basically anywhere that nerves exist that aren't in the CNS.

Then imagine the PNS trunk itself divides into smaller branches. One of those branches is a part of the PNS called the autonomic nervous system (ANS). As the name implies, the ANS does things automatically, without thinking, like breathing and heart rate and blood pressure. And off the ANS branch there is another very special part of the nervous system—your gut's nervous system—called the enteric nervous system (ENS, and that's the last acronym, I promise).

The ENS is your digestive system's nervous system. The ENS is special. The ENS can operate autonomously from your brain. But the ENS is also in constant, direct contact with your brain.

That's because the ENS is made up of neurons embedded in the walls of our digestive system, from the esophagus to the anus. The ENS communicates through neurotransmitters. And there are five times more neurons in the ENS than in the spinal cord—about half a billion.

The ENS is often called "the second brain" because of its independence from the brain and because of this neural network's influence over the brain. The ENS not only receives messages from the brain; it sends messages back from the neurons acting independently all along the digestive tract.

Remember that neurons, which are found in both the gut and the brain, are shaped differently from the other human cells. Neurons have a bumpy, rootlike structure. The place where a root from one neuron meets a root of another neuron is called a synapse. Most synapses are "chemical" synapses, meaning that they use chemicals (neurotransmitters) to transmit information between neurons. Some neurotransmitters are produced in the gut, as we've discussed, and are impacted by the types of food you eat.

Messages sent from the ENS influence brain plasticity, neurotransmitter production, and even behavior. You may perceive something as fair or unfair, stressful or not, depending on the messages your gut sends your brain (remember the *Cyberball* experiment). And those messages can change depending on your food.

THE VAGUS NERVE

The vagus nerve is a bundle of nerves that physically connects the digestive system directly to the brain. It's a cranial nerve, meaning a nerve that enters and exits directly through skull openings. There are only 12 of these cranial nerves. The vagus nerve is unique among cranial nerves in that it's a two-way highway (much like the ENS)—it sends information both from the brain to the gut *and* from the gut to the brain.

We know that the vagus nerve is important for mood regulation. In studies, mice will push a lever for stimulation that goes directly to their vagus nerve, showing that vagus-nerve stimulation gives some sort of pleasure or reward independent of other sensory cues. Vagus nerve stimulation alone can increase dopamine in mouse brains.

Stimulating your vagus nerve can be calming—a centuries-old technique called the Alderman's itch involves massaging your ear just above the ear canal to promote relaxation. We now know that the outer ear directly connects to the vagus nerve. Stimiluating the vagus nerve is currently an FDA-approved method for treating depression and has proven anti-inflammatory properties. The vagus nerve is also activated during mindfulness training.

The vagus nerve is a major focus for food–mental health researchers. It has a lot of receptors, and studies are geared toward characterizing all these receptors. We know that some receptors on the vagus nerve's fibers match the molecules for the signals your gut microbes send out. Scientists are trying to understand that matching system better because there might be a way to block the transmission of signals that cause depression or anxiety symptoms right at the synapse.

Researchers have cut animals' vagus nerves to see the effect on mood and the brain. Remember the studies about how effective helpful bacteria can be in regulating stress? Well, researchers tried replicating those studies, but this time cut the vagus nerves in the mice. When the vagus nerve was no longer connected to the brain, the beneficial bacteria *Lactobacillus* didn't work to reduce the stress response. Additionally, when the vagus nerve was cut, the body's ability to make new neurons was hampered. And each neuron can create up to 40,000 connections, so it's important to keep them.

Furthermore, the vagus nerve endings communicate with your gut microbes using enteroendocrine cells (the "sensory cells of the gut"). These enteroendocrine cells in the gut lining act on the vagus nerve fibers to help release signals sent by your gut microbes. Enteroendocrine cells in the gut can communicate with the vagus nerve in 100 milliseconds, which is faster than blinking.

Neuroscience historically has looked more at the brain's cortex (the four top fingers of the hand model of the brain), where high-level conscious functioning happens. Research on the vagus nerve's importance has also increased interest in the brain stem. Neuroscientist Mark Solms writes in his book *The Hidden Spring: A Journey to the Source of Consciousness* that the brain stem is itself a densely tangled core of nerves and is "where consciousness arises; it is the hidden wellspring of the mind, the source of its essence." By not looking at the brain stem, we potentially neglect the basal, driving forces of emotion, pleasure, wishes, and desire that the vagus nerve attaches to.

We're pleading with our rational minds to stop eating cake when it's potentially a whole other part of our brains that drives the impulse of *more cake*.

To reiterate, the ENS and vagus nerve are food-mood mechanisms that are affected by factors other than the gut microbiome. And there is a lot of ongoing research about which structures in the body connect the gut and brain, in addition to the ENS and vagus nerve. That research will likely continue well past our lifetimes. So how can we help ourselves now? One way is to improve our eating patterns to support our gut microbiomes.

Using Food to Support Your Gut Microbiome

Think of the digestive system as a factory that processes raw materials—food—into something your body can use for energy and nutrients. And think of the microbes that the food comes in contact with along the way as some of the factory's highly specialized workers. There's a lot going on all over the factory, and these highly specialized microbial workers exist all along the production line. But toward the end of the line, there is a room where most of the microbial specialized workers gather to team up in groups to do things that workers in the other parts of the factory couldn't do. Your large intestine is that room, where microbes create substances from our food that the body otherwise could not make.

Even if the factory's mechanics work really well, the quality of what you get out of it depends on what you put into it. A factory that has the best raw materials will have the best chance of creating a great final product. As microbes break down food, they produce metabolites (meaning, literally, by-products of metabolism). The metabolites affect the brain at the top of the central nervous system and can affect our emotional wellbeing. Metabolites can travel through the bloodstream to everywhere in the body; it's essential that half of the small molecules in your blood right now are products of bacteria.

A factory that has quality raw materials is also likely to attract other highly skilled workers who can work in tandem with the existing staff to create the best products. They help each other do things that none of them could do alone.

Eating food containing beneficial bacteria—fermented food like yogurt—gets some of the food's beneficial bacteria into your large intestine. Most of the food's microbes don't stay in your large intestine forever, but they do work with the bacteria that live all along the digestive system to improve what your body is able to make from your food. So fermented foods can contain both quality raw materials and specialized gut workers—a double benefit.

Different microbes make different substances, trigger different genes, and use food differently. Our food affects hormones and neurotransmitters, our hormones and neurotransmitters affect our feelings and emotions, and our feelings and emotions affect what we eat. It's another way that everything in the body is connected; it's a system and it can be circular.

To illustrate: The gut is an important regulator of cortisol and blood sugar. We've seen that cortisol is both a cause and effect of heightened fear and anger. High or low blood sugar can affect mood both short and long term; high blood sugar, for example, reduces the hippocampus's ability to react to stress. Better raw materials lead to better substances lead to greater emotional wellness leads to greater ability to thoughtfully choose raw materials.

There is a lot we don't know about how this gut-brain connection happens. But we know that improved food intake and eating patterns— better raw materials—are associated with improved mental health. Which kinds of microbes we have inside of us, and how many, are highly influenced by the food we eat—and there is research showing that the food we eat may be influenced by which microbes we have. Because the body is a system, the connections are both circular and complicated.

Diversity is the strength of any complex ecosystem. Generally, the greater the diversity of beneficial microbes in your gut, the stronger your gut is. Several studies show that more diverse gut microbiomes are associated with better health outcomes. And gut microbiome diversity depends in part on your eating patterns.

Some research is looking into whether specific types of bacteria are beneficial or not; if researchers found one bacterium that will make us better, we could all just figure out how to get more of that one bacterium. This is the lure of "superfoods"; that if we eat enough, say, spinach, everything will be fine. But that's not how microbial diversity works.

Tryptophan—an amino acid found in oats, nuts, cheese, and (famously) turkey—is essential for us to eat because our bodies can't produce it. Once tryptophan is ingested, different microbes do different things with it. Some microbes turn tryptophan into serotonin, which is then stored in the gut. But other, non-beneficial microbes turn tryptophan into a substance called kynurenine, which causes inflammation and has been implicated in psychiatric disorders. This is why you can't just say "eat more tryptophan." How the nutrients we eat are processed by the body is influenced by the microbes we have, which is influenced by what we eat because it's a system. And it's why we likely won't be able to create a superpill anytime soon that replicates all the gut-microbiome benefits of whole foods.

A study by the American Gut Project showed that people who ate 30 or more plant foods each week have more diverse microbiomes than those who ate 10 plants per week. According to microbiome researcher Rob Knight at the University of California, San Diego, diversity of plant intake has a stronger association with diversity of gut microbiome than recent antibiotic use. Antibiotics can be like a factory fire, burning many of the specialized workers in its path. Antibiotics can be necessary and lifesaving sometimes; we should just know that after the fire, you have to do some special planning and care to get the factory going again, along with working toward a goal of fewer fires.

Diversity is the goal, not some idea of a "perfect" gut microbiome, which doesn't exist anyway. Global research shows that people eating diets rich in whole foods have more diverse gut microbiomes. People living in nonindustrialized nations have more diverse gut microbiomes than people in industrialized nations. And lower diversity in your microbiome is linked to general inflammation, which—as we'll discuss in the next chapter—can influence emotional wellness.

There is so much ongoing research—about different kinds of bacteria, how they work together, their effects. But we know that gut microbiomes respond to dietary intervention. What we know now, and is actionable today, is that eating a diverse, whole foods diet helps diversify the microbiome.

Two recommendations for supporting your gut microbiome are eating foods with probiotics and prebiotics. "Probiotics" is a term describing bacteria that, when eaten, are beneficial for gut health. "Prebiotics" describes certain kinds of compounds that we eat. Prebiotics feed the good microbes that are already in your gut so those microbes can work even better. You may have heard of both probiotics and prebiotics because they've become something of a health trend over the past decade as research has piled up about their benefits.

PROBIOTICS

Probiotics are certain edible strains of bacteria that science has found to be particularly beneficial, for your gut. And "probiotics" covers hundreds of different species of bacteria, all in different combinations depending on what kind of fermented food you eat. Each probiotic is a living organism, each with its own unique genetic makeup. When you see labels on food or supplements, probiotics are measured in colony forming units (CFUs), which are usually in the billions.

Probiotics are highly beneficial, but the good bacteria in the food we eat don't usually wind up permanently populating our gut microbiomes. Most probiotics we eat pass through the gut microbiome like transient workers. By cooperating with the resident workers—the microbes that live in your gut—the transient probiotics in food encourage the resident workers to stay, multiply, and create a better working environment that creates better substances.

It's not like you eat yogurt and then the probiotics in the yogurt automatically live inside you. Probiotics don't usually replace the bacteria that are already there. But probiotics do hang out a while in your large intestine and, while they're there, they eat and digest and create metabolites, all of which are highly beneficial for the microbes that *do* live in your gut full time.

Fermented foods are particularly helpful as they can contain "active live cultures," a phrase you may have seen on the side of a yogurt container. Fermentation is the natural process of bacteria breaking down sugars (any kind of sugar, including the naturally occurring sugars in fruits and vegetables). The bacteria can occur naturally in or on the food, be added, or come from the surrounding environment (no matter how clean your kitchen is, there are lots of microorganisms in it).

During fermentation, the bacteria in the food change in quantity and type. Fermentation produces other substances, including different bacteria. Turning milk into yogurt produces beneficial metabolites like lactic acid that are ready before the food even hits our mouths. When cabbage is fermented, the resulting sauerkraut has way more lactic acid bacteria than cabbage does. The beneficial bacteria stay in the food and go into our digestive systems.

I wish probiotics were a one-and-done kind of remedy, but microbiomes are built up through eating patterns, not by eating yogurt one day and feeling like you're cured for life. A healthy gut microbiome is something you feed every day. And because gut microbiomes are unique like fingerprints, the effect of a probiotic on you—how your body reacts and whether the probiotics pass through quickly or set up camp for longer in your gut—will differ from others.

But the microorganisms have to be alive to get health benefits, and labeling laws currently allow listing of CFUs that are dead too. Your best bet is to find probiotic foods in the refrigerated section of your grocery store and keep them in the fridge at home. This is because, to keep all the beneficial bacteria, fermented food should not be pasteurized after fermentation; therefore, it's not shelf-stable.

Compare this process of fermentation to pickling. Fermentation and pickling are both ancient processes to preserve food. But for our gut microbiomes, fermentation is usually preferable because fermentation allows more beneficial bacteria to flourish during the process.

Forget for a second that we often refer to pickled cucumbers as "pickles." "Pickling" describes a specific process; "fermentation" is a process that is a type of pickling, but not all pickled foods are fermented foods.

Some types of pickling use vinegar; fermenting does not. This is partially because vinegar kills other bacteria—you've probably heard of vinegar as an excellent cleaner. There is no way to selectively kill only bad bacteria, so pickling with vinegar may also kill a lot of beneficial bacteria.

Vegetables pickled with vinegar will likely not have the same array of beneficial bacteria as vegetables fermented with bacteria in and around the vegetable. Vinegar pickling is great for long-term storage of food and can be really delicious. Vinegar pickling is not the enemy, and vegetables pickled with vinegar probably contain some beneficial bacteria, particularly if they are made with raw apple cider vinegar (which itself has a lot of beneficial bacteria)—all vinegars are not created equal.

But when you're considering gut health, fermentation is the way to go. It can get confusing—because fermentation is a subset of pickling, you can buy fermented "pickles." In the last chapter I'll give some practical pointers about buying fermented food.

For now, remember to choose foods where good bacteria can live until they get to their final destination—your gut. So it's likely that any food labeled as fermented and full of beneficial bacteria will:

» Be refrigerated;
» State that it is a fermented food; and
» State that it contains live and active cultures—maybe even specific strains of bacteria.

Let's look at what this means for, say, cottage cheese. There may be 20 kinds of cottage cheese at your grocery store. Ones that are made with vinegar—which many popular kinds are—are not fermented. But cottage cheese can also be a fermented food, made by adding bacteria to milk. If your cottage cheese is made by fermentation, it will likely say it on the package because fermented foods are so in demand these days. The package will also likely list some bacteria as ingredients because they were used to ferment the cottage cheese. And I've found that fermented cottage cheese has a pleasurable tang often missing in other cottages cheeses.

Fermented foods are worth searching out. In addition to the studies already mentioned about the connection between fermented foods and emotional wellness, researchers have found that people who have high microbial diversity also had a decrease in inflammatory markers, particularly when they eat a lot of fiber. Which makes sense, as we know that microbes love to eat fiber. And that brings us to prebiotics.

PREBIOTICS

A microbiome's gotta eat. And what it eats is prebiotics, compounds in food that help beneficial microbes to flourish. Prebiotics are not digestible by humans, so they make it to your large intestine undigested. As you may recall, this is where most of the gut microbiome action happens. For a long time, scientists thought that the main job of the large intestine was to process waste because it's where all the indigestible parts of food go. Now we know that microbes in the large intestine do a lot with your "waste" during digestion. In the large intestine, microbes convert prebiotics into substances that can support wellness.

Your microorganisms, the workers living in your large intestine, adore prebiotics. Microbes munch on prebiotics, producing beneficial metabolites like short-chain fatty acids that our bodies can't produce without the right raw-material foods. And when short-chain fatty acids are released into the bloodstream, they can reduce inflammation and support emotional well-being.

The best example of prebiotics is soluble fiber, found in foods such as onions and garlic. "Soluble" fiber just means that the fiber can dissolve in water. Human cells can't digest soluble fiber, so your microbes eat them. Science has identified other prebiotics, but soluble fiber has the most research. When we eat prebiotics, we feed our beneficial gut microbes. In a 2021 study involving 1,323 participants with PTSD, participants who consumed an average of two or three fiber sources each day showed fewer symptoms of PTSD. When participants in another study were given prebiotics, they showed lower levels of cortisol during a stress test and focused more on positive information than those who were not given the prebiotic.

The good bacteria in our microbiomes also support mental health by protecting the lining of our intestines. The intestine lining acts as a barrier between whatever is in the intestine and the blood circulating outside the intestine. Remember, there are things in our digestive system that we absolutely do not want to leak into our bloodstream—food molecules and bacteria, to name two—and our intestinal walls keep it all contained.

(When toxins do leak out, it's called leaky gut syndrome, which you may remember from Cryan's early research is associated with mood disorders.)

Toxins from the intestine that leak into the blood can cause inflammation in the brain, as we'll see in the next chapter. One way to discourage toxins from leaking into the blood is to have a strong intestinal lining. If you don't have enough good food—prebiotics—for your gut microbiome to feed off, the microbes will hungrily eat your gut lining instead. When the microbes eat the lining, the lining weakens and becomes more permeable. This is how toxins can leak out.

So prebiotics both allow your gut microbes to make substances that support mental wellness and help you maintain a strong intestinal lining, which further supports mental wellness.

Fiber is amazing, and you're probably not getting enough. Only 7 percent of Americans get their recommended amount of fiber (14 grams per 1,000 calories). It's tougher to get prebiotics into our diets when we eat ultra-processed foods. When food is refined, the fiber is stripped from grains to make flour. That's one reason that whole foods are so important for your gut microbiome. Researchers say that our gut microbiomes now are very different from the way they were when our hunter-gatherer ancestors subsisted on foraged foods. Some researchers believe that gut microbiomes today are dramatically different from even 75 years ago, as the ultra-processed food system now produces more processed food devoid of the fiber and nutrients generally provided by whole foods, which the good bacteria need to flourish.

Because food is one of the fastest ways to change our microbiomes by introducing new and beneficial microorganisms into our bodies that can affect how we absorb the rest of the food we eat, we need to focus on our eating patterns for emotional wellness. If you eat "perfectly" for one day and then give up, your microbiome will likely change for only several hours; what we need is an altered eating pattern, one that feeds the micro-biome what it needs daily.

"There is nothing coming up in the next few decades that will be better therapy than diet," says gut microbiome researcher Emeran Mayer at the University of California, Los Angeles. "With one foot, you're in the most cutting-edge science that has ever been done. The other foot is in the most traditional health recommendation."

You can go to a pharmacy and find a whole mess of prebiotic and probiotic supplements, some specified down to the bacterial genus and stamped with a weight-loss claim (the claims are, incidentally, not approved by the FDA). Or you can make it easy on yourself, your budget, and your gut by choosing to eat fiber and fermented foods.

The Fiber Gap

Our fiber deficiency has become so pronounced that nutrition scientists came up with a name for it: the fiber gap. Closing your fiber gap can support your emotional well-being and general physical health too.

Part of the problem is that we aren't eating plants in any version of their original state. Dietary fiber is found only in plant foods. And the ultra-processed foods that make up such a large part of our diets have little fiber—even those that are plant-based. This is one of the ways that food advice gets complicated: 100 grams of fresh corn kernels have about 3 grams of fiber, but after that corn goes through industrial processing, it can have as little as zero grams of fiber. However, both fresh corn and processed corn can be listed on an ingredients list as "corn." (And even when the fiber is left in after processing, the high heats involved in ultra-processing can destroy other nutrients and can change the molecules in corn, making the two chemically different substances.)

If we choose to do nothing else for our health (and, honestly, we all have some days like that), increasing fiber intake and closing our personal fiber gaps can have enormous benefits. Fermentable fiber—also known as soluble fiber, the type that our microbes love best—is essential for emotional well-being. Fermentable fibers are eaten (aka metabolized, fermented) by our gut microbes, and the by-products of metabolism are chemicals, such as fatty acids, that serve the human body well.

In one recent study, mice developed metabolic syndrome (including diabetes and high cholesterol) when given a high-fat diet. But when fiber was added to the high-fat diet, many of the problems associated with metabolic syndrome decreased or disappeared. The mice were found to have vastly different microbiomes after eating fiber, changes associated with better health outcomes. (One of my favorite things about this study is that it refers to "diet-induced obesity," recognizing that obesity generally is a complex condition that has to do with more than just food.) And remember that, in mice, hungry gut microbes that don't get enough fiber (through you eating fiber) will eat away at the gut lining.

Potatoes have fermentable fiber; fries don't. Root vegetables have fermentable fiber; and when root vegetables are fermented, they can have twice the fermentable fiber. But some insoluble fibers are fermentable fibers, too, so it may be best to focus on increasing overall fiber instead of splitting hairs.

Why and How to Be a Fiber-vore

1. Fiber can significantly slow absorption of sugar. When you're choosing food with some sugar but no fiber, consider either starting with fiber or adding in a food with fiber (nuts in candy, for example).
2. Some snacky ways to get fiber (that won't feel like you're eating the fiber version of what you really want to eat) include popcorn, guacamole, dipping vegetables, high-fiber bread, pumpkin seeds, crunchy baked chickpeas, almonds, and raspberries.
3. I personally can't believe popcorn isn't a more popular snack—it may have just gotten a terrible reputation because of artificial butter toppings and low-quality microwave popcorn. Instead, try buying a bag of loose popcorn kernels, place about a quarter cup in the bottom of a large microwavable bowl and seal the top of the bowl with microwave-safe plastic wrap. With a fork, poke a few holes in the top of the plastic and microwave the bowl for about 3 minutes, or until there is a second between kernels popping. This tastes better than any standard microwave popcorn, doesn't have added chemicals, and will save you money.
4. Choose beans or legumes as your protein. Half of a cup of lentils has 9 grams of protein; ½ cup of chicken breast has 15 grams of protein. But the lentils provide 8 grams of fiber, with all kinds of benefits that the no-fiber chicken breast doesn't have. This isn't about choosing lentils every single time unless you want to. It's about focusing on the benefits that variety can bring.

SHOULD YOU TEST YOUR MICROBIOME?

I gave some top microbiome researchers my gut microbiome test results, which arrived several weeks after sending my stool sample in. I was hoping, based on the company's ads, to find out which bacteria make up my microbiome and a list of specific bacteria and foods I should eat for optimal wellness.

It turns out that these tests are often losing the bacteria for the bacterium. Some are so focused on looking for a single specific bacterium, perhaps forgetting that many diverse bacteria work together as a system for a healthy gut microbiome. And a healthy gut microbiome is itself part of the complex system that is the human body. And that the body is part of the complex system that is emotional wellness. It's not as easy as taking a probiotic marketed to me by a company that already had my $400.

"None of those pills or probiotics or anything will in any way replace the critical role of what we do many times a day in terms of putting fuel into our body and the complexity of what that fuel does and how it works in our body. It's not even close," says nutritional psychiatry researcher Felice Jacka. "You're talking about these thousands of bacteria; you're talking about very complex methodologies that we're only just beginning to get right. In the meantime, people can just get on with having a healthy diet that will best support their microbiome to do all the things that it does to influence their health and metabolic processes and the way their genes express themselves."

"It's understandable that you want to get your microbiome tested," microbiome researcher Turnbaugh assured me. "As long as you do it with the spirit of discovery, not absolute solutions. If you get your microbiome tested, we don't even know what to do with that information."

"A lot of people assume that if you have a microbiome profile it's predictive," he continued. "But most of the things you're measuring in those profiles are bacteria that are largely unstudied. We don't really know very much about what they're actually doing in the gut or why, at a more molecular, cellular level, they matter for disease."

The technology of gut microbiome testing is ahead of what you can actually do with most of the information you get from having your microbiome tested. I ordered one kit that came with a tape measure and asked me to send my waist and hip measurements, which seemed like a cheater's way for them to recommend some sort of fat-loss microbiome thing even if my actual sequencing didn't show whether I was overweight.

And in some cases, Jacka told me, two companies analyzing the same sample of gut bacteria could come up with very different reports about what microorganisms live inside you. That's because companies use different methods of testing and have their own different genomic "libraries." Each library contains fragments of DNA from each type of microorganism. They compare your sample to their own particular library to identify which microorganisms call you their host.

"You might get a completely different set of data by applying one library compared to another library. You're not going to get the same results," said Jacka.

For me, about half of the bacteria in my test were classified as "unknown."

"These results are considered normal," the test stated.

Also, a gut microbiome test represents a snapshot in time—a person's microbiome changes regularly, as we know. And some medicines, like oral antibiotics, wipe out about a third of bacteria in your gut microbiome until it has time to repopulate through food, environment, and the many other things that impact the makeup of your microbes. (There is research showing an increase in depression in people who take antibiotics that doesn't exist when people take antiviral medication or antifungals.)

Printed in large letters on the results of my test was the legally required statement that gut microbiome test kits are not considered diagnostic and are not approved by the Food and Drug Administration. Your doctor likely will have no idea how to read your microbiome test if you hand her a printout. It can be hard to swallow for a precision-health-data-hungry society that the best intervention we have is still the ancient remedy of eating. But feeding your gut microbiome quality food is one of the best ways to be a good host.

Every single researcher I spoke with said we are at least years away from the kind of personalized gut-microbiome nutrition that some companies offer. In the meantime, evidence supports a whole foods diet, fiber, and fermented foods for gut health.

You can save your $400 or spend it on health-supporting foods. No need to have a test done to support your microbiome. Just look at what you do three times every day.

Tangy Herb Butter

Remember that cooking fermented food kills many of the beneficial microbes. That's OK though, because this recipe takes something we love, butter, and adds yogurt to give it a smooth tang—and, in the process, the butter gains beneficial microbes. It's a delicious spread for toast or tossed with fresh peas or other vegetables. Winning all around.

Butter combined with other ingredients—herbs, spices, sun-dried tomatoes—is called compound butter. Swap out the thyme and garlic for other herbs and spices you love. (One of my personal favorite compound butters is a salty honey-cinnamon.)

MAKES ABOUT 1 CUP

4 tablespoons softened butter
1 garlic clove, minced
1 tablespoon chopped fresh thyme
¼ teaspoon salt
⅓ cup Greek yogurt

In a food processor or in a medium bowl, mix the butter, garlic, thyme, and salt until combined. Pulse or stir in the yogurt until combined. Refrigerate until desired consistency.

CHAPTER 4

Inflammation

---

*"Holding on to anger is like grasping a hot coal with the intent
of throwing it at someone; you are the one who gets burned."*
—BUDDHAGHOSA

EMOTIONAL WELL-BEING'S CONNECTION to inflammation and the
brain can be surprising to some who went to medical school decades
ago. For years, the prevalent idea was that the membrane surrounding the
brain, called the blood-brain barrier (BBB), protected our brains from all
the toxins circulating in our blood. Remember that the nervous system—
with the brain at the top—is the body's high-speed communication system
and is critical for our survival.

Blood is the body's slower-paced communication system, using hormones that circulate to other parts of the body. At any given time, our
blood may be carrying waste products, carbon dioxide, and a number of
compounds related to the immune system and fighting infection. These
toxins can damage the brain if they can get to it.

But many physicians believed that the brain was completely protected
from blood toxins through the BBB. The foundation of this belief was a
series of experiments in the early twentieth century to see where blood toxins can travel in the body. Researchers injected blue dye into an animal's
circulatory system. The animal's internal tissues all turned blue—except for
the cerebrospinal fluid in the brain and spinal cord. Researchers believed
this meant that the body has an impermeable barrier to protect the brain

from blood toxins (such as dyes). Then, several years later, another experiment showed that dye injected into cerebrospinal fluid turned the brain and spinal cord blue, but not any other part of the body.

For decades the conventional medical wisdom was that the central nervous system was compartmentalized from other parts of the body through the BBB. The body wants to protect the brain, its master controller, so the BBB is a strong level of protection. Scientific consensus back then was that the body had an impenetrable boundary between our brains and our toxin-rich blood. So even when there were a bunch of pathogens bouncing around in our blood, the brain wouldn't be affected because those pathogens would knock up against the BBB and never make it to the brain.

Then, in the mid- to late 1900s, better technology showed a more accurate picture of the BBB. The BBB exists, but it's not as impenetrable as scientists had believed. There are several areas of the brain where the BBB is weak at best, allowing many substances to pass back and forth. And the BBB may be at its lowest, allowing pathogens into the brain and potentially affecting our emotions and mental health, when our bodies experience inflammation.

The Immune System and Emotional Well-Being

Inflammation comes from your body fighting something that the body perceives as potentially harmful. The body fights threats through the immune system, a network of defenses that includes some of your organs, cells, tissues, and chemicals that your body makes. When the immune system detects a threat, it calls up its resources—the parts of the immune system—to address the threat.

One immune system resource your body uses is your white blood cells, which are the body's soldiers in the war against infection. Blood can get to most parts of the body, so blood cells are an effective way to travel. But when a lot of blood goes to one area of the body due to a perceived threat, that area has a lot more happening in and around it than before the threat arrived. And the body reacts to these increased resources: blood vessels get larger so more blood can come into the area. Because there is so much blood in one place, the area swells and gets warm or hot to the touch—a phenomenon commonly known as inflammation. This is your immune system at work.

Here's a pretty straightforward example of how it works: You fall and cut your knee, and some potentially harmful bacteria get into your body through the opening of the cut. The immune system perceives the harmful bacteria inside the body and calls up its troops to go to where the threat is. In a properly functioning immune system with a common virus, the body uses its resources to destroy the threat. Your knee may swell, it may feel warm. That inflammation is your immune system working, sending resources to your knee to help heal the wound and fight the bacterial threat.

If you're thinking, *hmm, this sounds a lot like what happens to our bodies when we feel negative emotions*, you're right. The immune system effects of expanding blood vessels and areas feeling warm or hot are also ways our bodies respond to emotions. That's because the release of cortisol—which can happen when you're afraid or angry—activates the body's immune system and can cause inflammation. This can be really helpful when we need a rush of blood to quickly run away from a threat.

As an acute stress response, inflammation is fantastic because it means that part of your body is healing through resources rushing to the area that needs help immediately.

But chronic inflammation—constant activation of the immune system—can be a huge health problem. Our body's automatic responses and the world we live in today are a mismatch. Today, threats often do not require the cortisol our bodies produce to help us escape—you can't run away from traffic, quizzes in school, or meetings with your grouchy boss.

And to make things worse, modern threats are everywhere and constant. When our bodies go through the physical effects of stress often, we can have chronic low-grade immune system activation. And chronic immune system activation often means chronic inflammation, which can create damaging changes to the brain. Because chronic inflammation anywhere in the body, it turns out, has effects that can permeate the BBB.

We know now that the BBB is not a solid barrier; it's made up mostly of cells that are tightly packed together, meaning that certain small molecules—including molecules that can be toxic to the brain—can make their way to the brain. It's not impenetrable; it's semipermeable. So the BBB is not as protective as doctors previously believed.

And it's true that most blood vessels in the brain are safe within the BBB, protected from toxins circulating throughout the body. It's also true that the only way molecules can get into the brain is if they somehow bypass or pass through this barrier (which is both good and bad news, as it's tough to get the large molecules of antioxidants and potentially beneficial antidepressant drugs through this barrier).

But research shows that inflammatory compounds in the blood (which can be triggered by food, as we'll see in a minute) can break the BBB and cause inflammation in our neural cells that directly impact mental health. The chemicals that immune system activation and inflammation send circulating through the blood can damage the brain.

One side effect of inflammation is increased cytokines in the blood. Cytokines are a group of substances that are a by-product of the immune system's process, including inflammation. Until recently, neurons were thought to be protected from cytokines by the BBB. Now research shows that at least some cytokines can pass the BBB and spur brain inflammation. Also we now know that there is no BBB in some regions of the brain—for example, in the circumventricular organ of the hypothalamus, which regulates mood, emotion, and appetite.

Inflammation can actually change how the brain operates and our emotional well-being, as a host of scientific evidence shows:

> » Less inflammation can lead to more and healthier neurons. Research shows that inflammation may affect neurogenesis, or the creation of new neurons and other brain cells. Furthermore, in overfed mice, the brain's immune cells—known as microglial cells, which ususally clean up dead neurons—can start eating live neurons.
> » Depressed people have higher levels of interleukin, a cytokine that reflects how inflamed our bodies are.

» When people take antidepressant medication, one frequent result is less body inflammation.

» One study shows that children who had physical inflammation at nine years old were more likely to be depressed at eighteen.

Increasingly, research shows that chronic inflammation and depression have a bidirectional relationship, that inflammation often occurs in people with depression, and people with depression often have high levels of inflammation. We don't know to what extent inflammation causes mental health issues, or mental health issues cause inflammation, or both—it's a bit of a chicken and egg problem—but we know the connection is there. As an international group of nearly thirty researchers wrote in a 2019 article, "One of the most important medical discoveries of the past two decades has been that the immune system and inflammatory processes are involved in not just a few select disorders, but a wide variety of mental and physical problems."

We know that when your body constantly addresses threats, it can experience constant inflammation. And one thing that can constantly threaten and inflame, or soothe and calm, the body is food.

Emotions and Inflammation

Emotion researchers have grouped all our emotions into foundational human emotions based on extensive research spanning decades. Foundational human emotions are ones we share across cultures, geographies, and time based on factors like universal facial expressions and effects on the body. Psychologists debate the exact number, but there are likely somewhere between four and seven foundational human emotions. The Pixar movie *Inside Out*, which animated the emotions going on inside an adolescent girl's mind, used research to settle on five emotions for its main characters: Joy, Sadness, Anger, Fear, and Disgust. Without getting too into the ongoing debate, some psychologists claim that disgust is a subset of fear, leaving four foundational emotions: mad, sad, glad, and scared.

It's helpful to categorize our feelings into the four foundational emotions because it can make it easier to identify what we're feeling, to then understand what's happening inside our bodies in response to that emotion.

These physical effects of emotions happen across races, ethnicities, and borders to prepare our bodies to act in response to how we feel. Of course, what triggers the emotions can vary widely, given each individual's different experiences. Recognizing your emotions can help you understand what is happening in your body and help you use the science of emotional eating in your everyday life. Your emotions can alter both what your mind wants and what your body needs, and you can eat in a way that satisfies both.

There is compelling science that your body needs more of certain nutrients when you're in certain emotional states—more magnesium when you're stressed, for example, and zinc when you're sad—which we will discuss in more detail later. But it can be harder to make those food choices when you're in an intensely emotional state. Research shows that people feeling emotions they perceive as negative are more likely to make health-supporting food choices *if* they thought the negative feeling was fleeting. And other evidence shows that the ability to come out of a negative emotional state is likelier if you make certain food choices. Again, we see that the food-emotion cycle can be vicious or virtuous.

Eating for emotional health can do the same thing. It can help you be mad but not hostile, to be glad but not boastful, to be scared but not paralyzed, to be sad but not disconsolate. And that resilience is underpinned by the knowledge that how you feel right now is not how you'll feel forever. The ability to process emotions as they arise, without retreating from reality, creates a path for a better overall mood in which life's inevitable problems won't determine your sense of self.

SCARED

Fear is our emotional reaction to a threat. As with other emotions, fear can be based in the actual moment (you're about to take a test), experiences you had previously and are projecting onto the moment (one time—maybe even a long time ago—you failed a test), or from both. Here's a look at how the feeling of fear works in the nervous system.

Let's say you are at home in your backyard and you hear something that sounds like a gunshot. The noise releases vibrations into the air. Those vibrations reach your ears and go to your brain, which perceives it as a sound. The amygdala might jump to attention to start the fear process because all it senses is "loud, threatening, gunshot-like noise." The cortex might then apply past learning to the fear—maybe you remember that you live next door to someone who has a car that constantly backfires, and it sounds like a gunshot.

Or maybe you have past experiences with gunshots, or the best explanation given the circumstances is someone shooting a gun near you—in which case your body produces energy to fight it or flee it. The amygdala controls fear and the fight-or-flight response. So if there is a perceived danger, the amygdala sets a bunch of things into motion. When the amygdala is activated, it tells another part of the limbic system, the hypothalamus, to tell the pituitary gland to make hormones that will help the body react to fear, something called the adrenocorticotropic hormone (ACTH). The pituitary gland shoots hormones out into the bloodstream.

One effect of all that ACTH is that your body releases cortisol, which raises blood sugar and white blood cells (which fight infection)—in other words, it increases resources to react to the threat that caused your fear. Hormones also dilate the pupils to take in more light to fight a threat. Your heart beats faster to circulate more blood to the legs for your flight response and sends less blood to the not-as-immediately-important stomach and skin (goosebumps are in part your skin trying to warm itself when blood has been redirected to other parts of your body, causing the muscles at the base of each hair follicle to contract). Blood flows toward your limbs, meaning there is not as much going toward your heart. The logic centers of the brain back off as the amygdala, which runs on instinct, ramps up.

The fight or flight response is useful when coping with physical danger, but unhelpful when trying to keep it together in the office. There is actually a third option in addition to fight or flight, which also really doesn't help with our symptoms: freeze. Kent Berridge, the researcher mentioned earlier when discussing how babies react to sugar, has experimented with fear in rats. In one setup, when the lab rats hear a tone, they know they will get a foot shock and there's nothing to do about it, so they remain frozen in fear. As Berridge puts it, when the rats see that the universe is against them, they just freeze. And then you're not using any of those fear resources your body created.

Many of the things that cause fear in us these days don't require physical fighting or fleeing. Fear comes from the unknown, and these days there is a lot we don't know, from age-old problems like pandemics and terrorism to modern ones like cyber-trolling. We sometimes consider reacting to a current danger using tools that may have served us in a previous—but different—danger. But our bodies stay in a state of high alert unless we do something to change it.

In addition to cortisol, when you feel fear your nervous system tells your adrenal glands to pump out another hormone, epinephrine—otherwise known as adrenaline, which we covered in Chapter 1. Adrenaline has some of the same effects as cortisol: increased heart rate, increased blood flow to your brain and muscles, and higher blood sugar. When your adrenal glands are activated, your body also needs more vitamin C. And humans are one of the few mammals that can't make their own vitamin C.

In healthy young people, stress is associated with a temporary decline in the function of the layer of cells that line blood vessels, known as the endothelium. This decline is likely because of the widening of blood vessels during stress to accommodate for the increased blood flow that comes along with the stress hormone adrenaline. Evolutionarily, when your body feels stress, it produces adrenaline for more energy so you can physically run away from something—because the threats used to be physical— think of the old "chased by a saber-tooth tiger" reference. In a small sample of twenty-one healthy young people, eating two butter croissants during times of stress further decreased vascular functioning when compared with a group that did not eat butter croissants. The high amount of fat may interfere with the body functioning under stress, and then with the body's recovery when the stress is gone.

Fear also affects how we taste, as the inflammation that often comes with it can shorten the life span of taste cells. Stress generally alters taste receptors. Under stress, our hedonic response to sugar is heightened, probably because of the energy it gives us to fight the stressor. When we are scared, we eat high-density (high-calorie) foods that fuel the immediate need for more energy to replenish the resources that our bodies are using in being ready for a threat. Reduced taste sensitivity can increase sugar and salt preference. In one study, when people were stressed, they rated bitter flavors as more bitter and sweeter flavors as less sweet. This effect was pronounced in "highly arousable individuals," or people whose temperament or mood was generally stressed.

Some foods that are helpful in coping with fear include citrus fruits, yellow peppers, kale, broccoli, brussels sprouts, and strawberries. Also try cooking techniques that are meditative and include a visual accomplishment—cleaning and chopping can be really satisfying. I get a lot of pleasure from prepping this sheet pan recipe, which has a rainbow of ingredients that cook on their own, then combine beautifully in a dinner bowl.

Sheet Pan Dinner

Sheet pan dinners have everything on one pan, cooked in one oven, at one temperature, that's all done at one time. It's great for when you're dealing with a lot—those times when takeout sounds way more relaxing than cooking. There's just enough chopping involved in prepping the vegetables to get you involved but not so much that it becomes tedious. And pounding chicken with a rolling pin gets out some extra energy.

SERVES 2

Extra-virgin olive oil
2 boneless, skinless chicken thighs
¼ cup tahini
¼ cup plain Greek yogurt
2 tablespoons lemon juice

continued

1 garlic clove, minced

Kosher salt

1 lemon, sliced into thin rounds

1 (15.5-ounce) can chickpeas, drained

1 yellow bell pepper, sliced into ½-inch-thick strips

2 cups broccoli florets

1 medium carrot, sliced into ½-inch-thick rounds

4 ounces Brussels sprouts, quartered

½ teaspoon paprika

Heat oven to 400°F and line a baking sheet with parchment paper or foil.

Place the chicken on a cutting board, cover it with plastic wrap, and hit it with a rolling pin several times, just to make it uniformly thick and even.

In a small bowl, whisk the tahini, yogurt, lemon juice, garlic, and a pinch of salt.

Brush both sides of the chicken with oil and season with salt. Put the chicken on one side of the baking sheet, slather with a quarter of the sauce (reserve the rest for serving), and top each thigh with a couple of slices of lemon.

Rinse and dry the chickpeas and put them on the end of the baking sheet opposite from the chicken. In between the chicken and chickpeas, place the pepper, broccoli, carrot, and Brussels sprouts. Drizzle ¼ cup of oil over everything and sprinkle with salt. Sprinkle paprika on the chickpeas.

Bake for 30 minutes, until the chicken is cooked through. Serve with the remaining sauce.

MAD

Anger is an emotional response to a perceived injustice. It is a discrete emotion but has physical effects similar to fear. Anger, like all emotions, begins with a stimulus, either internal or external. A lot of people, including me, spend a lot of their lives trying to get rid of stimuli that could cause anger—leaving unhealthy relationships with certain people, turning down the news, avoiding crowds. This can be helpful. We can work in our lives to reduce the number of anger situations we get into.

Unfortunately, you can't get rid of all the stimuli that produce anger. If you have a family of any type—parents, children, siblings, people you love so much that you'll never get rid of them even though they have little traits that drive you bonkers—anger is unavoidable. Simply by caring and loving, critical human endeavors, you will feel anger no matter how self-actualized you are.

In a world that isn't fair, in which people who deserve good things don't get them and those who we feel don't deserve good things have mind-boggling wealth, anger can become a constant undercurrent in our lives. There's no shortage of injustice in the twenty-first century; our bodies could stay in an anger reaction permanently.

That would not be ideal, as anger also uses a lot of your body's resources. The body responds to anger with its ancient fight-or-flight system to have energy to fight the source of your anger. Someone takes your share of the antelope you just killed, so you get angry and force them to give it back.

When you're angry, your amygdala is activated, as it is with fear. Your glands release cortisol and adrenaline, which allows you to do physical things to fight the injustice that you otherwise couldn't do. Your immune and digestive systems slow so your body can send all its resources toward fighting. As with fear, anger raises blood pressure, increases heart rate, and creates muscle tightness and tension. Blood sugar increases.

Norepinephrine (also known as noradrenaline) and epinephrine (also known as adrenaline) are released, just as with fear. Sometimes we feel hot when angry, as body temperature can rise in response to our higher heart rate and more rapid breathing. Your blood goes toward your muscles so you can fight, taking resources away from digestion and metabolism.

But excess cortisol can cause the neurons all over your nervous system to weaken, damaging them to the point that the neurons can die. This happens especially in the hippocampus and prefrontal cortex, which leaves you with literally fewer brain cells, causing memory problems and brain fog.

And all that cortisol can reduce serotonin production, which can further negatively affecting well-being and mood. Decreased serotonin is associated with aggression as a response to angry feelings. And angry outbursts are also linked to depression. Both repressed anger and raging outbursts are associated with heart disease. During the two hours after such an outburst, you are three times more likely to have a stroke from a blood clot to the brain or to have brain bleeding.

It's a system that used to be well suited to human life but can be a mismatch with how we experience anger today. It's hard to express anger in an office or in front of kids, and there are limited ways to get out the physical energy that anger can bring.

Some foods that can be helpful in managing anger are cold-water fatty fish (tuna, salmon, anchovies), pumpkin seeds, beans and lentils, and leafy greens. Foods with calming smells like lavender or rosemary are good, too. Try out some physically exerting cooking techniques that may help use up some of the energy hormones flooding your body—whisking, kneading, and grinding are great.

Salmon Cakes

If you're fish-curious but you don't want to invest in a fresh salmon fillet that may sit in your refrigerator for days until you're motivated enough to make it, try canned salmon. Canned fish can be delicious, especially when combined with fresh herbs, bitter lemon, and crunchy crumbs.

My recipe calls for nut crumbs. Nut crumbs are a great alternative to bread crumbs. You can buy them prepackaged in the bread crumb aisle or make your own: grind nuts in a coffee grinder until they resemble bread crumbs. My favorite combination of nuts for crumbs is pistachios, almonds, and cashews.

You can make these as two big cakes, or four to six smaller cakes if you like crunchy, delicious ugly bits. I once made fish cakes and was eating the leftover crunchy bits out of the pan because I was worried they were too ugly to serve. Then I noticed other people swooping in to eat them too. So I put them all on a platter and slapped a label on it that said "delicious ugly bits," which are sometimes the best part of fish cakes—and life.

MAKES 2 CAKES AS ENTRÉES OR 4 TO 6 CAKES AS APPETIZERS

2 (5-ounce) cans salmon, drained
1 egg, beaten
1 tablespoon nut crumbs or bread crumbs
2 tablespoons plain Greek yogurt
1 tablespoon chopped parsley
1 tablespoon lemon zest
Kosher salt and freshly ground black pepper
1 tablespoon extra-virgin olive oil

In a medium bowl, combine the salmon, egg, nut crumbs or bread crumbs, yogurt, parsley, lemon zest, and a pinch each of salt and pepper. Pat the mixture into cakes—two larger cakes or four to six smaller cakes.

In a skillet, heat 1 tablespoon oil and fry the cakes over medium heat for about 4 minutes per side. Serve warm, over salad greens, with vinaigrette drizzled over the top.

SAD

Sadness is the emotional response to losses, big and small. Everything we put in our lives serves some sort of purpose, and when it goes away we need to grieve the loss, even if it's the loss of something that didn't benefit us or that we never really had.

Sadness changes the body, and the way individuals respond to or express sadness runs a wide spectrum. As children, we learned that a frowning person with a fat teardrop rolling down her face was the symbol for sadness. But sadness is one of the most vexing of human emotions because it manifests so differently in everyone. Unprocessed sadness can manifest as unusual behavior, irritability, or low self-esteem. Sadness can be a peculiar struggle because many of its coping mechanisms involve detachment from life, which only tends to increase sadness. And unaddressed sadness can lead to anxiety or depression disorders. That's especially relevant, as many of nutritional psychiatry's studies about food and mental health focus specifically on anxiety and depression, which are also the two most prevalent mental health issues today.

But try telling any of this to a person who is sad. For many of us, the biology of sadness doesn't matter in the moment. Over the span of two years, I had six failed pregnancies, followed by three failed IVF cycles (this kind of heartbreak is possible, timewise, if you try hard enough). After deciding to end the game of "let me see if I run into this wall again; maybe this time it won't hurt," after all the injections and disappointments and so many times squinting to see if there was a positive line on the pregnancy test, I felt deep, engulfing, terrible sadness. It was the kind of sadness that you climb out of inch by inch, but only if you choose to grieve. But I'm not great at asking for help. I had been around so much chaos when I was a kid, I recognized the no-win sadness as a familiar place. It was an attachment to something that didn't benefit me.

When we're sad, the amount of inflammatory protein in the blood increases and, as we have seen, that inflammation is associated with lower mental health outcomes. You can get sore muscles and headaches from the increase in inflammatory proteins. When you're sad, your blood pressure decreases. Sleep is disrupted. Your immune system lets its guard down. Studies show that small, simple projects like cooking can help with sadness by offering us a sense of accomplishment from creating something. Cooking isn't always relaxing—especially when others rely on you to feed them—but you don't have to make a showstopping dish. Focus on small, rote, easy tasks, which can be almost like meditation.

Some foods that can help: dark chocolate (if you're not a fan, look for bars that have cocoa butter listed as an ingredient, as this can have a creamier texture that milk chocolate fans will like), hot peppers, eggs, and turmeric (use this spice liberally). Keep it simple when choosing what to cook; research shows that small achievements can bring big, improved mood changes—but even the smallest setback can crush you when you're already sad.

Dark Chocolate Peanut Butter

Some food writers roll their eyes at three-ingredient recipes, but I've written a lot of them and sometimes three ingredients are just magic. You can easily remember what to buy at the grocery store—no phone-scrolling through a recipe needed. Even when life is crazy and I can't even with the cooking, I can motivate to throw three ingredients together.

Plus a big part of eating for emotional well-being is being realistic about what counts as a win, depending on what's going on in your life. Aspiration is great but when you're already sad, it can be particularly difficult to move the goalposts.

Also . . . dark chocolate and peanut butter? You'd have to pay me not to make this. It's a great way to sneak your way up to dark chocolate if you're used to eating milk chocolate.

MAKES ABOUT 1½ CUPS

2 cups (about 10 ounces) shelled, roasted, and unsalted peanuts
1 cup dark chocolate, chopped or broken into small pieces
Kosher salt

Place the peanuts in the bowl of a food processor and run the processor about 2 minutes—the peanuts will grind, then stick together, then turn into a ball, then turn into peanut butter.

continued

Add the chocolate and run the processor until chocolate is incorporated, about 90 seconds (time will depend on the size of your chocolate pieces).

Taste and add salt to your liking (I put in 1 teaspoon, but I love a salty peanut butter).

This is amazing served as a dip for apples. It will thicken in the fridge.

GLAD

You won't be surprised to hear that there are many positive health conditions associated with being happy. Serotonin is elevated, cortisol decreases. In several studies, people with higher happiness levels over time have lower incidence of heart disease. Happiness is positively associated with the strength of your immune system. Happiness can lengthen our life spans and make our years better while we are alive.

Gladness is a resource. Just as resilience comes from experiencing difficult times, we can use happiness to fortify our emotional selves. When you're glad, it's easier to make choices that improve your eating pattern, which can make it easier to manage thoughts that can get in the way of your flourishing. Eating to support mental health while you're glad is like a love letter to yourself that you mail today and get in a week when you really need it. It's happiness management.

Yet the most successful people I know have some issues with the happiness that comes when positive things happen. I've seen lots of anger-management classes and stress-management classes and depression-management classes. There should be joy-management classes too, and cooking mental-health-supporting food and feasting with others would be big parts of that class. Gladness feels good, so it's sometimes accompanied by fearful concerns about what will happen next, whether our happiness is sustainable, or how others feel about our happiness. Gladness can feel precarious to those of us for whom it's sometimes fleeting.

When you're in a happy state, it's easier to make choices that improve your eating pattern. Childhood food memories are powerful, so powerful that they are markers for what our comfort foods are now. We don't choose our happy childhood memories any more than we choose our childhood microbiome. But we can work on creating our own comfort food.

We forget that we teach ourselves to eat every single day. Creating our own food memories means eating particularly well when we are happy and have a window of opportunity to create happy associations with food that will help our long-term wellness.

Foods to focus on: oysters (if you don't like them raw, try grilled), leafy greens, nuts (especially Brazil nuts). Make something in a big batch that can serve lots of people you like and that can be frozen for times when you aren't in a cooking headspace. I call these surge capacity dinners, and they are perfect for happy times.

Easy Grilled Oysters

Oysters can be intimidating; there are so many kinds that it can get confusing. If you're thinking there's no way you're going to shuck oysters at home, try this recipe instead. The next time you're grilling, throw a few oysters on the grill. Don't worry about choosing the right kind, just get started.

MAKES A DOZEN OYSTERS

**1 dozen fresh oysters in the shell
Kosher salt**

Make sure all oysters are clamped shut (discard any that have opened on their own). Rinse the oysters in cold water.

Turn the grill on medium to high heat. Place the oysters curved side down directly on the hot grill. Close the grill lid and let oysters cook for 4 to 5 minutes.

Open the lid—the oysters will open when they're done (discard any that don't open after 5 minutes). Place the open oysters

continued

on a platter, making sure to keep any liquid inside the shell. To keep the oyster shells from tipping over, place each shell on a small pile of kosher salt.

Loosen the oyster meat from the shell with a knife and slurp the oyster right out of the shell. Great by itself or with a dot of tangy herb butter, a squeeze of lemon, or dash of hot sauce (or all three).

The Immune System, Food, and Emotional Well-Being

When the food we eat on a regular basis damages our health, we are constantly putting our immune systems on high alert. And the immune system and the gut go hand in hand. The lining of the gut is home to 80 percent of all immune cells in the body, and their job is to decide what is friendly and what is a foreign object that they need to fight off. When the immune cells in the gut malfunction, the whole system can go haywire. The gut can interpret some foods, commonly dairy or glucose, as invaders that need to be fought off—this is known as a food allergy. That threat brings blood to the area, causing inflammation.

Inflammation can occur in other, more common ways than food allergies. It happens much more often than you might think. Remember that when we don't eat enough fiber, our good gut microbes, which really want to eat fiber, will turn to eating our intestinal wall lining. That weakened intestinal wall can let things that are inside the intestine—and should stay there—into the bloodstream, sometimes causing leaky gut syndrome. That's bad enough.

But even worse, it's a compounding problem because in response to weakened intestinal walls—which are their own problem—your immune system kicks in to help, causing inflammation. That inflammation may be able to address the acute problem of stuff from the intestine leaking into the bloodstream, which is great. But when we have an eating pattern that doesn't include enough fiber on a regular basis, there can be chronic immune system activation, which can lead to chronic inflammation.

As we've seen, chronic inflammation is associated with poor mental health. And there is a strong indication that diet can improve mental health through its effect on inflammation status.

In a 2021 meta-analysis, researchers found a link between what they call the Dietary Inflammatory Index (DII) and mental health. The more inflammatory one's diet, the higher association with symptoms of mental disorders.

What is an anti-inflammatory diet? It's the same kind of diet that has been tested for improving poor emotional and mental health: a Mediterranean-style diet with a special concentration on whole foods, fermented foods, and fiber. It's that vicious or virtuous cycle again—we eat poorly, our bodies become inflamed, and our brains can suffer, which can cause us to eat poorly; or we eat mood-supporting foods and our bodies are not as inflamed and can potentially support our mental health.

Another consideration is the oxidative stress that poor nutrition can cause in the brain. Free radicals are unstable atoms that can harm cells from the inside out by, for one, damaging DNA within a cell. And we know what damage to cells does—calls up the troops of the immune system, causing inflammation. Free radicals happen to all of us as we age, as oxidation is a normal physiological function. But poor diet can speed up the creation of free radicals. The more free radicals bouncing around your body, the likelier your cells will take a beating.

Oxidative stress is a chemical reaction that happens when your body's cells produce more potentially harmful substances, such as free radicals, than the cells can handle. It can be caused by diet—when you eat refined sugar, the spike in your blood sugar floods cells with sugar, which gives quick energy but promotes oxidative stress. Evidence shows that people with depressive symptoms often have higher levels of oxidative stress markers.

Inflammation anywhere in the body can affect emotional wellness. And what we eat can have a direct impact—negative or positive—on our inflammatory state. In a 2018 article reviewing the social behavioral effects of inflammation, the authors found that "research points to an important role for inflammation in shaping social processes."

Blood Sugar

Evidence increasingly shows that blood sugar is a vitally important metric that few people pay attention to. I wear a continuous blood sugar monitor, as I have an unavoidable autoimmune condition known as type 1 diabetes.

Type 1 diabetes was known as "juvenile diabetes" until the late twentieth century, when young kids also began developing type 2 diabetes, a condition which has the risk factors of excess weight and low levels of activity. These factors are increasingly common in children, and in the dearth of activities available to non-sports-star kids. In type 2 diabetes, the body makes insulin, but the body's use of insulin is confused.

For people with type 1 diabetes, the body simply doesn't make insulin at all (or makes very little) because their body kills the pancreas's insulin-making cells. No one knows why the body attacks itself—this is what happens with all autoimmune conditions. It's estimated that less than 5 percent of all diabetes in America is type 1, although no one is sure, in part because America's diabetes statistics don't differentiate between types.

I have a nearly undetectable, quarter-sized monitor attached to my upper arm at all times, telling me exactly what my blood sugar is, and whether it's going up or down, on an app connected to my phone. Right now it's 129 and trending down. Blood sugar, also known as blood glucose, is critical. If you have low blood glucose, your body can't function—the few times my blood glucose has gone low, it feels very suddenly as if I can't think. I slur my words, and don't make sense because the brain runs on glucose, so if the brain doesn't get glucose, it doesn't function properly. Sometimes I break into a cold sweat, a reaction from muscles not getting glucose either. I know I have to get a little sugar into my system immediately because that is what gets blood sugar to go high really quickly—also known as a blood sugar spike. In the case of a type 1 diabetic, it goes from a dangerous low—perhaps 50—to a stable level, say 100.

The reason that orange juice spikes blood sugar is that it's almost totally pure sugar, with nothing to slow it down. In contrast, a whole orange eaten as a piece of fruit has fiber in it from the flesh of the fruit. If I eat an orange, my blood sugar goes up more slowly because the fiber is preventing the sugar from hitting my bloodstream all at once. In people without insulin-related conditions, this process is regulated by your pancreas releasing insulin (the human body adjusts to conditions with amazing flexibility). For the rest of us, we have to think through it—our brains are our pancreases. With a piece of fruit, my blood sugar is a steady up and a steady down. Personally, I drink juice only in low-blood-sugar emergencies (the app on my phone dings if I go below 55). Or in cocktails—alcohol in most forms lowers blood sugar because it keeps the liver otherwise busy with processing alcohol's mild poison. (The liver is where the body stores extra glucose and, in case anyone needs to hear this, heavy alcohol use is not a suitable long-term treatment for high blood sugar.)

Everyone processes food differently. Rolled oats—not maple sugar–flavored but just oats—for some reason spike my blood sugar in a way that oats don't affect others I know with blood-sugar monitors. I am 100 percent certain that no one will ever figure out the mechanism for my higher blood sugar on oats, no matter how long I live. I still eat oats (yum); I simply use the knowledge of what they do to my specific body. So I eat oats before I do cardiovascular exercise, which lowers blood sugar significantly.

Individual bodies react differently to all kinds of substances in foods. And bodies don't always act how you may expect. Insulin, for example, is secreted by the body to process sugar. But a small single-blind study of fifteen healthy adults, published in 2023, found that a beverage containing artificial sweeteners results in higher insulin levels detected in saliva—just as sugar-sweetened beverages do.

As mentioned earlier, increasing fiber can also slow the absorption of sugar, so it's often best for blood sugar steadiness to eat some fiber with a sugary food. This is popularly known as "food sequencing"—an unfortunately "pop-diet," suspicious-sounding name for something that is basic nutrition science. Eating a bunch of candy followed by a bunch of broccoli will likely spike blood sugar higher and more quickly than eating broccoli followed by that same amount of candy. That's because if your stomach has some fiber in it already, it slows the absorption of sugar from the candy.

In studies of people with type 2 diabetes, those who ate fat and protein before carbohydrates had lower long-term blood sugar and released naturally occurring GLP-1, an active ingredient in injectable weight-loss drugs like Ozempic.

This is both the wonder and frustration of the human body. We don't know why bodies react differently to many things. It's the goal of the precision medicine industry to give personal recommendations down to your specific cells, but it does so with varying degrees of reliability. Listening to what's happening in our own bodies, a skill known as interoception, is tough to cultivate. But I've paid so much attention to my blood sugar over the years that I can often tell where my blood sugar is just by how I feel physically (and not just when it's dangerously low). My experience is supported by a 2023 study showing that mindfulness training improves interoception and eating foods that support emotional well-being.

Low blood sugar can be a problem for both type 1 and 2 diabetics because—although there are approximation formulas to guess how much insulin your specific body needs at a specific time—every body is different and every moment can be different, even for the same body. Recent statistics show that people who are food insecure are at a greater risk for hypoglycemia (low blood sugar) events. During the one-year study, 1,000 adults with diabetes were followed over 12 months. About 200 participants said that they skipped meals or cut out eating because there was not enough food, and half of those suffered a severe low blood sugar event.

Low-or high-blood sugar can damage the body, which activates the immune system, which often leads to inflammation. A recent study found that adhering to the Mediterranean diet reduced the incidence of type 2 diabetes in participants with high risk for cardiovascular problems.

Weight

Let's talk about weight. I know, I don't want to either, but there are a lot of people seeking meaning in either the bottom of a pint of ice cream or a smaller pair of pants (sometimes both). There is science linking higher body weight with inflammation and a less diverse gut microbiome, which, as we've seen, can cause all sorts of issues.

Since all the science unfortunately gets filtered through diet culture, the damaging popular opinion is that weight is infinitely malleable, that a "perfect" weight is a sign of virtue. When we focus on weight, we can lose sight of the goal of eating patterns that support mental health rather than only a lower weight.

There is much more to learn about potential causes of higher body weight. Jeffrey Gordon runs one of the most prestigious microbiome labs in the world at Washington University in St. Louis. (Microbiome researcher Peter Turnbaugh went through the Gordon Lab before he started his own.) One of the Gordon Lab's most significant studies used the microbiomes of human twins—one overweight, one thin—to populate the gut microbiomes of mice. The mice were then fed the same diet and the same number of calories. But the mice who had received the microbiome of the overweight human twin gained more weight and had higher body fat than the mice who received the microbiome of the thinner twin.

Researchers took it a step further and transferred different types of bacteria into overweight mice's microbiomes, then saw those mice's body weight decrease. Research went on to show that when overweight mice were given a diet that resembled a Western-style diet, they gained more weight even when they were exposed to lean-human microbiomes.

Anyone who has ever tried to lose weight knows that it is more complicated than eat-less-exercise-more. High body weight is an energy imbalance, but that energy balance depends in part on what your body (and your gut microbes) does with the food it takes in and how much energy (calories) you get from it.

It's unscientific, simplistic thinking that weight is always due to someone eating uncontrollably, even though that is a popular idea in our culture. And those of us with any excess weight can internalize that maybe there *is* something wrong with us, and the resulting stress can exacerbate whatever inflammation we might have from excess body weight.

Assigning vice or virtue to people by their weight (confident and trust-worthy for people who meet popular body ideals; lazy, dumb, glutton-ous for people who don't) does not motivate weight loss or greater health. Some studies show that weight stigma actually worsens health by increas-ing emotional distress, which is a precursor for depression, anxiety, and disordered eating.

In a recent international study of 14,000 adults, participants often incorporated weight stigma into their own internal narrative, what they say to themselves in their own minds, a phenomenon called "weight bias inter-nalization." This study showed that "the more people internalized weight bias, the more they had gained weight in the prior year, used food to cope with stress [we can assume in an unhealthy way], avoided going to the gym, had an unhealthy body image, and reported higher stress."

Internalizing weight stigma seems to be a warning sign for all kinds of physical and emotional issues. And telling someone that you feel bad about your appearance can be embarrassing, adding an extra obstacle to seeking support to deal with the stress of internalizing weight stigma.

For a terrific depiction of weight bias internalization—and the running commentary that can happen in our own minds about our weight and others'—the Apple TV+ series *Physical* re-creates that internal dialogue. "You're nothing. You're a ghost. A fat ghost," the narrator, an aerobics instructor, tells herself internally while acting pleasant and cheerful on the outside.

When I started studying the food-mood connection, I had some con-cern that the science-backed connection between food and mental health could lead to blaming a person with depression for their own problems ("eat better, you'll be fine") as popular culture often does with weight stigma. Food can be part of the solution if you want to change either your mood or your weight, but science tells us that both are complicated and multifaceted. Channeling before/after, fat/thin narratives (she finally stopped eating and lost the weight!) promotes the idea that weight and emotional well-being are both final destinations, when they are really jour-neys. And shaming your higher-weight or emotionally distressed self is unhelpful when it comes to health improvement. Studies show that weight stigma often prevents people from being physically active. And we know that lower physical activity can increase inflammation in people of all sizes and that even a small amount of mild exercise can help alleviate symptoms of depression and anxiety.

It's so strange to me that today we have a phrase—"body positivity"—to describe not hating your body and not transferring your own fears about weight onto how you evaluate others' bodies. But that is the norm today. Even if we all ate and exercised the same every day, we would all be different weights and shapes.

We know from research that stress can decrease the quality of your microbiome, which can increase the possibility of weight gain. Stressing over weight loss is like diving into the ocean to stay dry. Humans have so many biological compensatory mechanisms to make sure that we eat enough but far fewer to make sure we don't eat too much. Our bodies evolved to deal with lack of food, not windowless grocery stores with thousands of ingredients in multiple permutations available 24 hours per day.

The current focus we have on body weight isn't working to decrease body weight or improve emotional wellness. Weight-loss diets often focus only on decreasing calories and give no attention to your microbiome, or inflammatory potential, or pleasure, which are all important, science-backed ways of improving emotional well-being. Weight-loss diets also often don't focus on the nutrient density of food (how many nutrients per calorie food has), which, as we'll see in the next chapter, is critical for emotional wellness.

The way you lose weight is calories in, calories out, but what happens inside you during the processing of your calories matter, too, in ways we are just beginning to understand. Inflammation can be a contributing factor to overeating because the signals that go from your gut to your brain that say you've had enough food can be disrupted by inflammation. Some researchers believe that ultra-processed food, because of its often-high simple carbohydrate, sugar, and unhealthy fat combination, messes with the signals the gut sends to your brain to say that it's full, so eating ultra-processed food is in itself a risk factor for weight gain.

In 2019, NIH researcher Kevin Hall was skeptical that processed food alone can cause weight gain. So he ran the first randomized, controlled study about the effects of ultra-processed food. It was a four-week study of 20 healthy adults. For the study, the participants were all required to stay at NIH's inpatient facility so NIH researchers could know exactly what participants ate for the entire four weeks.

Participants were randomly separated into two groups. For the first two weeks, group one ate a diet of ultra-processed foods and group two ate a diet of whole foods. Then the groups switched—for the final two weeks, group one ate whole foods and group two ate ultra-processed foods. They were given three meals each day and one hour to eat the meal, in addition to offers of snacks from whatever category—ultra-processed or whole foods—they were eating that day. Participants were told to eat as much or as little as they wanted. All the meals in both diets were designed to have the same number of calories, energy density, macronutrients (fat, protein, and carbohydrates), sugar, sodium, and fiber. An ultra-processed breakfast was, for example, a commercially mass-produced breakfast sandwich (turkey bacon, egg, and American cheese on an English muffin), tater tots, and orange juice. The whole foods breakfast could be scrambled eggs and homemade hash brown potatoes with an orange.

Each group ate more calories (an average of 500 more) each day they ate ultra-processed food, even though, in the other two weeks, they were offered the same number of calories in each meal that was made from whole foods. During the two weeks that each group ate whole foods, each participant in the group lost about a pound. During the two weeks a group ate ultra-processed foods, they gained a pound.

We'll talk more about other ways that ultra-processed food can interfere with emotional wellness through nutrient deficiency in the next chapter. But if you're concerned about inflammation caused by excess weight interfering with emotional well-being, avoiding ultra-processed foods is one way to address it.

Every researcher I interviewed who expressed an opinion about weight and diets said to focus on nutrition—which often comes in the form of whole foods. Focusing on nutrition rather than weight could be far more effective in getting the result you want—a flourishing life.

"The relationship of diet and nutrition and mental health seems to be quite independent of body weight," microbiome researcher Felice Jacka told me. "Forget about your body size; focus on the quality of your diet." Diet-culture mentality can often lead to an all-or-nothing way of thinking—I ate a handful of M&M's, might as well eat the whole bag. But research shows that eating for health is about an eating pattern, not being perfect.

"In the SMILES trial, people experienced a major change in their depression symptoms without changing their body weight," Jacka continued. "Most people in that trial were overweight or obese, and no one lost weight. That wasn't the point."

Amber Alhadeff, the hangry neuron researcher, told me: "I have a very anti-diet attitude because of the science. Eat what gives you pleasure because if you don't, that's where you run into trouble. I love eating fruits and vegetables, but I also like dessert. So I eat dessert every single day because I like it and it's an important joy I get in my life."

In other words, it is possible to improve mental health through food without focusing at all on body weight. To me, this is a revolutionary message in an industry that desperately needs a makeover. You and your doctor (choose your doctor carefully) can decide whether you want to focus on changing your weight, either up or down.

While there is an association between ultra-processed food and weight gain, we all know that one person who eats garbage and is still thin. People who do not have extra weight are not always eating whole foods. Focusing on whole foods rather than weight is both scientifically and emotionally sound.

Eating is intimate and personal, and even voluntary food restriction can cause disordered eating. I've earned this mindset the hard way. I had food withheld from me as a kid, depending on how big I was or how much money we had, and I still experience that sense of scarcity even as an adult. Making food choices is still a deeply ingrained celebration of my independent adulthood; sometimes when I'm stressed, I notice that the refrigerator is unusually full (of mental health–supporting foods, but still very full). In response to feeling insecure, I will buy more than I need to get the soothing feeling of being food secure. But one thing I've realized: We still hand down food neuroses as often as we hand down food traditions.

This is no one's "fault." It's not my fault for being taught these ideas about food as a child, and it's not the fault of anyone who taught me because that's what they knew at the time. But it is my responsibility now. And I am rewriting the story of my food life by focusing on getting the most out of food rather than fighting it. This in itself is an act of mental health self-care for me. Because negative body image is insidious—you feel imperfect and, even when you do lose weight, it's never enough.

Can you imagine if we lived in a world where, really, anyone overweight doesn't deserve love? Respect? Human kindness? That's a recipe for truly decreased mental health.

Eight Principles for Eating for Emotional Well-Being

1. We need pleasure every day. There is no RDA for pleasure, but you still need to make sure you have some.
2. It's a journey, not a destination, and we focus on progress over perfection. We work on our mental health every day; the same is true for eating. You get to do it all over again every day. You can see this as exhausting, or you can see it as freeing. I choose the latter.
3. Pay attention to fiber. If you really want something to count, count fiber grams. For most people, the more fiber you eat, the better.
4. Diversity is a strength. Diversify the types of plants you eat, even if it's just one bite.
5. When faced with a choice to eat alone or with others, we eat communally.
6. We are kind to ourselves about food. Our emotional well-being depends on it.
7. Flavor is created in the brain. Everything that we do around food preparation and eating matters.
8. We pay attention to our blood sugar. Food affects different bodies in different ways. Spiking and falling blood sugar can be a precursor for inflammation.

CHAPTER 5

Nutrients

"We are indeed much more than what we eat,
but what we eat can nevertheless help us to be
much more than what we are."
—ADELLE DAVIS

EATING TO SUPPORT mental health isn't a check-off-this-food-and-you'll-be-fine situation. That's the same wishful thinking as the pill mentality. "Take two walnuts and call me in the morning" doesn't work. Science right now is trending away from reductionist thinking (eat this nutrient or take this pill and be emotionally well forever) and embracing a systems method (food works with our bodies on multiple levels).

Evidence shows that, in addition to other evidence-based ways of addressing emotional well-being, an eating pattern helps—one that regularly includes a variety of nutrients, as well as pleasure, microbiome-supporting foods, and anti-inflammatory foods. The Mediterranean diet (and other similar dietary patterns, such as Okinawan and Norwegian) has large amounts of fruits, vegetables, whole grains, and anti-inflammatory fats, which have nutrients that are linked to improved mental health. Not surprisingly, all of these cuisines have cultures that celebrate whole foods as pleasurable.

Food and its compounds are extraordinarily complex; these compounds help your body process vitamins that you just can't get from a pill. You may avoid nuts because they are high in fat, but it's that fat that allows your body to absorb the other fat-soluble vitamins in nuts, such as vitamin E. The system works. We're just not using it properly.

Nutrients and pleasure can work together too. Your gut has receptors that can sense fat and send signals to your brain that it has experienced the sensation of fat. Researcher Amber Alhadeff calls this gut-brain connection "the sixth sense."

The Gut Sense

The gut sense that detects nutrients is influenced by the gut microbiome but is independent of it. As discussed in the last chapter, labs can breed mice to have no gut microbiome (this is not currently a research option with humans). Even mice that have no microbes still have a gut sense. And we know that nutrients in the gut activate the vagus nerve—remember that the gut microbiome uses the vagus nerve as a communication device too—because in mice, cutting the vagus nerve inhibits the effects of fat on the brain.

You've probably heard the saying "I feel it in my gut" referring to a feeling that has little basis in knowledge but is just something you know. And as we've discussed in previous chapters, the gut has its own neurons and its own nervous system that connect directly to the brain. Science can now show us that there is a gut sense. In her research, Alhadeff has shown that foods are sensed in the gut through the digestive system's receptors and transporters. And the gut communicates its contents to neurons in the brain that drive our behavior.

The gut sense reacts independent of any other senses related to the food—taste or smell or touch. In studies, the gut sense sends the brain messages about what kind of food it has in it, even when the food is injected directly into the gut—food that is not chewed and swallowed. The gut senses food in the absence of other senses being triggered as the nose responds to an odorant.

Remember the brain's hangry neurons, the ones that feel both hunger and anger, and stop being activated when we have food? In studies by Alhadeff and others, when mice have food placed directly into their stomachs, bypassing their mouths altogether, the hangry neurons are calmed equally well as when mice eat food through their mouths.

There are numerous other studies in mice showing that food injected directly into the gut, with a total absence of any other kind of sensory cues, activates a gut-brain food response that drives behavior. Here is an example: A mouse is introduced to two sugarless flavors. When the mouse eats one of the flavors, researchers inject an infusion of sugar directly into its gut (not into its mouth, so it never actually tastes the sugar). The other flavor releases no sugar infusion into the gut. The mouse will always prefer the flavor that gives the gut sense of sugar. It turns out we don't even need to taste the food for the gut to send reward notices to our brains. Also, when you inject food directly into the mouse's stomach, a dopamine signal is sent directly into the brain, even with no taste or smell or other sense involved. So, totally separate from our sensory experience of eating, there is a pure reward sense for nutrients that is driven entirely by the gut.

Sure, we like the way food tastes and we love the act of eating. But activation of sensors in the gut is a huge part of what makes food so rewarding to our brains. It's part of the reason why the chew-and-spit diet never works, and why food rich in sugar and fat is so rewarding.

Fat and sugar have different pathways to get to the brain. So when we eat a food that is rich in both fat and sugar, our brains may be flooded with pleasure signals from more than one pathway. That's especially important for humans because there aren't a lot of foods that are high in both sugar and fat that occur in nature—it's usually just one or the other (nature may have done us a favor with that). You really have to get to manmade foods to find the fat/sugar bombs of candy bars, pastries, even processed savory foods. This may account for some of the reason that the chef who lost the sense of smell still enjoyed Cinnabon, which is high in both sugar and fat.

Artificial sweeteners can really play with your mind. They do not send the same reward signals as sugar. We may taste almost the same things in our mouths, but you can't fool the gut. With technology that wasn't available even five years ago, we can now see immediate neural activity in awake animals as they behave, and see that artificial sweeteners do not give the same reward signals as sugar, nor do artificial sweeteners' rewards last as long.

"I think the gut sense is the most important sense for feeding behavior," Alhadeff told me when I visited her lab.

Nutrients and Emotional Well-Being

A nutrient is anything your body uses to survive, grow, and thrive. There are six main nutrients (or seven, depending on which scientist you ask): fat, protein, carbohydrates, vitamins, minerals, water, and—this is the debated one—fiber.

Dietary nutrients are divided into two categories. Macronutrients are nutrients your body needs in large amounts that provide the body with energy (calories): fat, protein, and carbohydrates. Micronutrients are nutrients your body needs in amounts smaller than macronutrients, a category including vitamins and minerals. A lot of vitamins are referred to by letter, making them as identifiable as the alphabet we learned as toddlers. (Which would you rather eat, vitamin D_2 or ergocalciferol?)

In the same way that you are a whole person, not just a collection of organic compounds, food is not just a collection of nutrients. Valuing food through a nutrient lens only and looking at food as simply the sum of its parts is known as nutritionism. For people who like eating, nutritionism is an unhelpful paradigm, simplistic at best and harmful at worst because it keeps us from pleasure. We've already seen that food pleasure is an important component of humans' relationship with food—but it's not easily measured on a scale to fit within a government-backed chart like the Recommended Dietary Allowance. You can't tell people that they need this many units of pleasure per day.

Nutritionism says yogurt is a combination of calcium, vitamin D, and the bacteria *Lactobacillus*. But the way you experience yogurt is a holistic experience—the creaminess in your mouth, the tang, maybe chunks of fruit—in addition to the nutrients. What do we talk about when we talk about nutrients? Gorgeously drippy ripe peaches, hot chicken soup, chewy bread, airy macarons, snappy string beans. Nutritionism loses the forest for the trees or, rather, loses the food for the nutrients.

There is evidence that nutrient deficiencies can contribute to development of mental health problems and make symptoms worse, so it's important to understand nutrients' significance. And increasing certain nutrients has been shown to improve stress response, depression symptoms, and overall mood in human studies. Additionally, there are certain nutrients that are required as precursors to creating neurotransmitters like serotonin and dopamine.

NUTRIENT CASE STUDY:
LONG-CHAIN OMEGA-3 FATTY ACIDS (DHA AND EPA)

In the next chapter you'll find a list of nutrients and foods that support emotional well-being to guide you through the grocery store or menu. To give you a sense of the kinds of research that go into the food-mood connection, we'll talk about one of those nutrients in depth here.

Remember that back in 2006, NIH researcher Joseph Hibbeln found that omega-3 fatty acids were associated with reduced aggression. He had already produced other reports on omega-3s; these studies arguably inspired and ignited the next two decades of research into the food-mood connection. In Chapter 6 we will discuss more than a dozen nutrients that are associated with improved emotional well-being, and each could probably be its own book. But omega-3s are a great introduction to the kinds of noteworthy studies being conducted and nuances that can help us understand how nutrients generally support emotional well-being. So let's get a little granular about omega-3s as an example of how nutrients can help.

All fats—butter, oil, the white streaks in a marbled steak—contain fatty acids as part of their chemical makeup. There are different types of fatty acids, identified by their chemical makeups. One family of fatty acids is known as polyunsaturated fatty acids (PUFA). Within the PUFA family there are two main types: omega-6 and omega-3. Within omega-3s there are three main types: DHA, EPA, and ALA. Of those three types, DHA and EPA, known as the long-chain omega-3 fatty acids, have the most evidence that they support emotional well-being. We'll get to how ALA (the short-chain fatty acid) can help in a minute, but for now we'll focus on DHA and EPA. So it goes like this:

FAT → FATTY ACIDS → PUFAS → OMEGA-3S →
LONG-CHAIN OMEGA-3S (DHA, EPA)

DHA and EPA are probably the best-researched nutrients to support mental health. Their benefits are numerous—to name just a few: they can promote sleep (by supporting melatonin production), decrease anxiety, and alleviate depression symptoms. Omega-3s protect the brain's hippocampus, which has been shown to shrink during times of anxiety. People with depression often have lower blood levels of DHA and EPA. In studies, depressed people who take a DHA and EPA supplement report alleviation of some depression symptoms.

DHA and EPA are the fats where the mental-health-boosting action is, with one of the strongest connections of nutrient to mood. It makes sense, as the brain's dry matter is constructed of 50 to 60 percent fat, and DHA is a major structural component. Additionally, you need to eat fat for your body to get fat-soluble vitamins (such as A, D, E, and K) from your food to your brain.

Despite the importance of omega-3s to the body, the body cannot create them. Humans must get omega-3s from food. We must eat them for our bodies to function properly, which is why omega-3s are called "essential" fats.

DHA and EPA are found in fatty fish, seaweed, and algae. And fish can't make their own omega-3s (fish . . . they're just like us). They get to be omega-3-rich by eating microalgae and by eating other fish who eat microalgae. The human eats the tuna, the tuna eats the herring, the herring eats the microalgae, passing omega-3s up the food chain.

Algae has more than 40,000 species, and some species have more

DHA and EPA than others. The amount of DHA and EPA is increased or decreased depending on several factors, including sunlight and temperature. Farm-raised algae can be tweaked to have more DHA. Algae-derived DHA is already prevalent in milk and other products that have become DHA-enriched in the past 20 years, as DHA research has deepened and shown many health benefits.

Dozens of clinical trials have shown DHA and EPA to have positive effects on people with depression. Researchers have been looking at a link for years, spurred on by statistics that depression and mood disorder rates are lower in countries that eat more fish. And an analysis of different studies—involving 150,000 people in total—found when people eat more fish they have a lower risk for depression.

Also, lest we forget: Fat is delicious. Fat provides food with taste, texture, and aromas. It lends its own flavor and is a conduit for and concentrator of other flavors. It luxuriously coats the tongue, helping flavor to linger after the eating is over. Fat is comforting, prolonging the pleasurable feeling of a full belly and releasing relaxing hormones like dopamine. It provides more energy per gram than protein or carbohydrates, meaning that evolutionarily, people who loved fat survived the hunting and gathering era.

Humans are wired to want fat—remember that the gut sense can tell us when we've had fat even if we don't taste it on our tongues. And on our tongues, it gives us pleasure. If we know how much we love fat, and if we know how much some fats can help our moods, we can use fat to our advantage.

Omega-3s perform several emotion-related functions in your body. All living things are made of cells, and cells have semipermeable membranes. Semipermeable means the cells' membranes—which are fortified and strengthened by omega-3s—allow nutrients to flow in through the membrane and let toxins out. At the same time, the membrane keeps cell functions inside. Healthy cell membranes are great gatekeepers of the entrance and the exit alike, and healthy cell functioning is the basis for all health, physical and mental.

The third main omega-3 we mentioned above, ALA, has a chemical composition called "short-chain," so it's known as a short-chain omega-3 fatty acid. ALA comes from plants like walnuts, flaxseed, and leafy greens. If you aren't eating enough fatty fish or algae, your body can convert some ALA into EPA and DHA to make up for some of the deficiency. (Remember, your body can't make omega-3s on its own; you must eat some omega-3s to have any omega-3s.) But every body's ability to produce EPA and DHA differs depending on things like genetics and gender, just as each human body is different. But on average, eating ALA is a pretty inefficient way to get EPA or DHA—only about 10 percent of ALA can be converted into its longer-chain cousins.

Most of us don't get enough omega-3s of any type. To make matters worse, most people eat an overabundance of the other kind of PUFA mentioned above, omega-6s. Omega-6s are not bad on their own, but we eat such large quantities of omega-6s that they've started to crowd out brain-protective omega-3s. One big reason is that omega-6s are abundant in corn and soybeans, two foods that are in lots of ultra-processed foods because they are inexpensive to grow. An ideal ratio of omega-6s to omega-3s is about two-to-one. Currently, nations with lots of ultra-processed food eat about a twenty-to-one ratio. And that imbalance can cause inflammation, which, as we've seen, is strongly associated with mood and emotional issues. We need to eat in a way to ensure adequate omega-3 intake.

You can actually see neurotransmitters travel faster in brains that are well nourished with omega-3s than in brains that are malnourished. Researcher Kuan-Pin Su in Taiwan sent me photos from his lab, taken with a cutting-edge two-photon microscope. You can see that less well-nourished brains have fewer connections to other neurons. We know that psychiatric disorders seem to be affected by small vascular changes in the brain. In Su's research, he created blockages in the blood vessels of rat brains. The rats recovered from the blockages when they ate omega-3s. Omega-3s may be both protective and healing.

MACRONUTRIENTS AND DECISION-MAKING

Dr. Soyoung Park in Berlin studies how the foods we eat influence our brains and, therefore, our decisions and actions. She devotes her career to decision neuroscience and nutrition, two fields that are, she has found, inseparable. Park didn't expect her PhD in neuroscience to lead to working in the mechanisms by which food affects thoughts. But in her extensive research, she has found that we can alter our brains enough through food to influence our decisions. And this association could go back to the first days of humankind.

As I got on a video call with her, I could hear her baby crying in the background. *Oh no!* I thought. *She must be so uncomfortable! A baby crying in the background—I don't want her to be embarrassed.* I projected all of my own former mom anxiety of having a baby crying in the background onto her and tried to put her at ease by saying, "Bring the baby in, let's see the baby, I love babies!" I was way over the top, compensating for the me that I was years ago, who felt as if I had to apologize for every way in which my life was not the same when I became a mother.

Park waved me away in the nicest way. "It's HIS turn," she insisted, waving toward the baby's father trying to calm the baby in the next room. And that's when I knew I loved Soyoung Park. She can have a baby in the next room and talk about her groundbreaking research and know that a father's place is taking care of his own kid—that's not babysitting, that's being a parent.

Park heads the Department of Decision Neuroscience and Nutrition at the German Institute of Human Nutrition. Like so many in the field of how food affects the brain, she stumbled into it by finding dramatic results made possible by new research technologies.

For Park, as for many researchers, the human body is "both fascinating and frustrating." It's a holistic system that is tough to study as parts separate from each other because all parts are so intricately entwined. So in 2018 she carefully designed a study to see if people's risk behavior changed with the food that they ate.

There were eighty-seven volunteers, and she brought each one in for two mornings, about two weeks apart. Each time she fed the participants breakfast, offering a large selection of different foods. Each time she would draw blood from the subjects before and after they ate breakfast. On one day, each item offered was balanced more toward protein than carbohydrates, and on the other day each item offered provided more carbohydrates than protein. Three hours after the subjects ate, they played a game in which they got to split a pile of cash (not bad work as far as research subjects go).

Here's how the game went. Subjects were told that there was a person in another room playing the game with them. (Spoiler alert: There was no person in the other room; it was the researchers the whole time.) That "person" in the other room, called the proposer, had a pile of cash and was allowed to propose how the cash should be shared between themselves and the subject. If the subject—with a belly full of carbs or protein, depending on the day—accepted the offer, then both people got the cash. If the subject rejected the offer, no one got any cash.

The study represents what researchers call a "social decision-making" problem, to answer questions like:

» How do we respond when we are being treated unfairly but still being arbitrarily enriched?

» How do we view our random, unearned fortune in relation to others?

» How do we view acceptable sharing of resources?

» What guides humans when choosing between options when we see ourselves being treated unfairly in favor of another person?

Our outlook on these questions shapes how we fit into our larger community and environment and how we negotiate relationships, and it can be a crucial marker of emotional wellness. They are also interesting philosophical questions as we work to make the world more inclusive and equitable. But because the study focused on the subjects' internal perceptions about a potentially neutral situation, it brought all their past experiences to bear.

Park was surprised by how changing breakfasts changed behavior. On the protein-leaning days, subjects were more likely to accept the offer and get whatever unearned cash they were offered—which was always less than what the "proposer" took. Their self-interest and logical thinking outweighed their sense of injustice or anger. On carb-leaning days, subjects were more likely to reject the offers, focused on the unfairness of the other person getting more cash even though that meant that no one got any cash. When the subjects ate carbs, their anger outweighed their own self-interest in getting at least some cash.

Protein meant the proposer and the participant got some money, even though it was unfairly balanced. Carbs meant no money for anyone.

One big clue emerged as to why this was happening: The amount that the subjects' behavior changed was proportional to the amount of the amino acid tyrosine in their blood. And the amount of tyrosine was directly proportional to how much protein they ate. The subjects who ate protein showed more tyrosine, which is a precursor for creating the feel-good neurotransmitter dopamine—meaning that when you have tyrosine, dopamine is able to follow. The tyrosine precisely predicted how much subjects' behavior shifted from the carbohydrate-leaning breakfast.

Food consumption predicted social behavior. And social behavior changed when the same person ate different foods.

This was mind-blowing for Park and created ripples in both science and anthropological circles. She wound up getting calls from researchers around the world, excited about her findings.

Some anthropologists published a commentary in the *Proceedings of the National Academy of Sciences*, using Park's research as the basis for an evolutionary theory of why food affects human emotions. When we lived as hunters and gatherers, the theory goes, we consumed a lot of protein because of the foods we ate. Humans couldn't store food at that time, so we shared with each other more, simply for group survival, because having a large group around you meant greater protection and power. Because of the benefits of living in large groups at the time, there was greater social pressure not to get upset if your neighbor got an extra bite of food. So during this time the body adapted to produce dopamine when we ate a lot of protein. We know now that having sufficient, but not too much, dopamine is critical for mental health.

The theory continues: When we evolved to an agricultural society that grew crops, the food had higher carbohydrate content. We learned how to store food. We now had private property, and social norms developed around our sensitivity to fairness. We created complicated legal systems to enforce these sensitivities, to punish those who violated them. So our bodies evolved (or devolved, depending on your point of view) to associate carbohydrates with a sense of possession. What's mine is mine and what's yours perhaps should be mine too.

I'm not sure humans will ever be at a point where we can definitively prove theories of our own social evolution in relation to our biology, so this may always be just a theory. Grand unified theories that explain everything are seductive because they make everything seem so simple and right, like when puzzle pieces finally lock into place. But maybe our biological evolution is in fact a puzzle whose pieces lock perfectly together, given that evolution means developing things that benefit us and shedding things that don't.

I asked Park whether her work, which she did not anticipate years ago would be about food or social evolution, has changed the way she eats.

"I like this question," she said. "I have more awareness, but of course if I'm having an emotionally hard time, I also eat a lot of rice. Whenever I talk about this study people get very excited, and one of the most frequent questions I got was, 'What should I give my wife in the morning so that we can have a good life?'" She paused and I gave an exasperated eye roll. I couldn't help myself.

"Take the baby!" I shouted, remembering Park's crying baby a few minutes earlier. "Tell them to take the baby and she'll be happy. It's not about food—just take care of the baby." I mean seriously, do people need science to tell them this? It's been true since the dawn of humanity. Before you do all kinds of food permutations to turn your spouse into a compliant person, just help them.

Park laughed, then confirmed that she is not recommending a protein-only diet to make someone accept your unfair offers. We are feeling, eating, and social beings. And better eating is about diversity and eating patterns. But she acknowledged that food can turn problematic now that we are in a time in history when food is created specifically to give us extra pleasure through fat and sugar. Eating whole foods and cooking, she noted, is not easy these days.

CAN'T I JUST TAKE A MULTIVITAMIN?

There's so much health information out there, it makes you wonder how humans evolved without chewable calcium chocolates or enormous pills claiming to have 100 percent of everything you need. The real answer is food. "It's as if each plant is a pill itself," gut researcher Emeran Mayer told me.

Of course, you can't get food pleasure from a pill. There is also some evidence that if we try to take these beneficial compounds in pill form, the molecules in the pills are too large to pass the blood-brain barrier, which can limit the effectiveness of a pill.

But, additionally, plants (unlike pills) have their own immune systems, and when humans eat plants, we also get benefits from them. Polyphenols are compounds (collections of molecules) that occur naturally in plants and are part of their immune system, defending plants against things like harmful insects or damage from too much sun. What's good for plants is good for humans, as we're now seeing that the polyphenols that protect plants can also, for example, protect humans from inflammation when we eat them. The rub, of course, is actually eating the plants, which most of us don't do enough of. And researchers aren't sure yet whether polyphenol supplements are as helpful as the polyphenols that occur naturally in food.

Each plant has different combinations of polyphenols. And there are thousands of polyphenols that we know of—maybe more—so the possibility of combinations in a single plant is staggering.

From the research we have, we know food and the human body have an amazing symbiotic relationship that we are just beginning to understand. Some polyphenols suppress harmful gut microbes. Some polyphenols act as prebiotics—food for beneficial microbes, who munch on polyphenols' large molecules, breaking them down so they can be absorbed by the body. That munching may not happen in the same way in pill form. The majority of polyphenols, about 60 percent, are flavonoids, some of which give plants different colors. You've heard the advice to "eat the rainbow"? That is because of, among other reasons, the different flavonoids you'll get from different plants. The nutrients can be complicated; the food isn't. And, in 2023, the CDC reported that 49 percent of American children do not eat a vegetable daily.

The Nurses' Health Study, which looks into chronic disease risk factors in women, showed that women who ate more flavonoids had lower rates of depression. Multiple studies show that fruit and vegetable consumption is inversely proportional to development of depression or anxiety disorders. But in 2022, the CDC reported that only 12 percent of adults eat enough fruit daily (1½ to 2 cups) and only 10 percent eat enough vegetables (2 to 3 cups daily).

I, too, want to have my cake, eat it, and then take a pill to make it like it never happened. But it's not possible.

Supplements are supplemental; they don't replace a health-supporting eating pattern. Some nutrients are better than others in a pill, particularly if you don't eat the kinds of foods that have them. DHA and EPA work in a supplement form if you never eat anything that comes from the sea. Zinc, magnesium, folate, and vitamin D have been shown to be more beneficial as supplements than other nutrients.

Researchers of the food–mental health connection say that generally supplements are not a substitute for the vitamins and nutrients you find in food. The evidence shows that it's not just the nutrients that matter—the mechanism that conveys them does too. Food brings with it fiber, thousands of polyphenols, and pleasure. You just can't replace that with a pill.

Processed Food

Processed food, as with mental health, is a spectrum. What is "real" food? How close to its original state does a food have to be to count as "unprocessed"? Many meat substitutes count as ultra-processed food. Even if the meat substitute is made from plants, those plants have been changed a lot from their natural state, so much so that they resemble meat. They are unrecognizable as plants.

A helpful, if not well-known, way to look at food processing when making eating choices is the NOVA scale (NOVA is its name, not an acronym). The NOVA ranking system was developed by Carlos Monteiro at the University of São Paulo in Brazil in 2009, the result of research into why sugar consumption was down in Brazil but type 2 diabetes and obesity were up.

The NOVA scale is what Kevin Hall used to create meals for the NIH study showing that eating ultra-processed foods results in greater calorie consumption. NOVA's classification system was adopted by the United Nations (a sign that it is helpful across cultures). The scale ranges from one to four, with four representing the most processed foods, ones which should not be part of a regular eating pattern to support mental health. The groups are:

GROUP ONE. UNPROCESSED AND MINIMALLY PROCESSED: Foods that have gone through no or little processing—for example, drying, crushing, grinding, pasteurization, roasting, boiling, or freezing. Minimally processed means that the inedible or unwanted parts of the food have been removed. The processing of the food is so minimal that the differences are "not especially significant," according to the United Nations. Any processing is to make the foods suitable for storage (like freezing or fermenting) or to make them "safe or edible or more pleasant to consume." Unprocessed or minimally processed foods are often used as ingredients in your kitchen. *Examples: pasteurized milk, edible parts of plants (leaves, fruit, seeds).*

GROUP TWO. PROCESSED CULINARY INGREDIENTS: This group includes substances obtained from the foods in group one through industrial processes like pressing, extracting, or mining. These foods may contain additives that prevent microorganisms from growing in them or that protect their original quality. *Examples: oil, butter, sugar, salt, syrup, honey.*

GROUP THREE. PROCESSED FOODS: Products created by adding group two ingredients to group one foods. *Examples: salted nuts, canned fish, fresh breads and cheeses.*

GROUP FOUR. ULTRA-PROCESSED FOODS: This group describes foods that are a combination of ingredients, most of which are ingredients for industrial use, and these foods are themselves created through industrial processes like chemical modification. These foods are often ready-to-eat but may also have culinary use as an ingredient (high-fructose corn syrup, for example). They also often contain additives. So look on the side of, say, a box of breakfast cereal or a frozen pizza. You will see ingredients that you don't recognize as things you yourself would cook with—those are ingredients for industrial use. These foods are designed to be highly profitable, palatable, and convenient, and are likely to replace food from groups one, two, and three. *Examples: mass-produced breads and pastries, packaged soup, margarine, soft drinks.*

There are other scales to measure the degree to which your food was processed, but NOVA is widely used. It's not perfect. Pasteurized milk is a group one food, even though pasteurization kills helpful bacteria. But milk pasteurization also kills harmful bacteria that can be prevalent in milk (some experts say it's far more prevalent in milk from large industrial farms), which otherwise can make people very sick or even kill them. And not all foods within a group are equally nutritious. Both honey and white sugar are group two foods, even though honey has potentially health-supporting properties that white sugar doesn't.

But the scale is still valuable, particularly because we turn to ultra-processed foods so often—Americans get an average of 58 percent of calories from ultra-processed food. And generally the wealthier a country gets, the more its citizens eat from group four. We've seen this, for example, in India and China in the past few decades. The increased consumption of ultra-processed foods is often attributed to less time to cook (or at least a more rushed lifestyle). In some places, ultra-processed foods are a symbol of wealth and abundance.

Diets high in ultra-processed foods—diets with an ultra-processed eating pattern—are usually more energy dense (higher in calories) and less micronutrient dense (fewer vitamins and minerals, including the ones that help with mental health). And eating from group four foods often means reducing consumption of foods from groups one, two, and three. So the more ultra-processed foods you eat, the more calories you consume and the fewer nutrients you get. Remember that Kevin Hall's NIH study showed that people who eat ultra-processed foods consume on average 500 calories more per day, even when offered the same amount of calories from whole foods.

Unless your diet consists of foraged food or only what you grow in and make from your garden, the world is more complicated than the black-and-white division of processed food versus unprocessed food. But it helps visualize why people with plenty of access to food can be malnourished, in part because of the reliance on ultra-processed food. The scale isn't perfect. But some days—whether because of time crunches or desires—instead of focusing on which group one foods are healthier than others, it's helpful for me to focus just on staying away from group four foods.

And group four foods usually come with food labels, which can be confusing if you don't know how to use them. Eating for emotional wellness doesn't mean examining labels in the ultra-processed food aisles to see which box has the most magnesium. This is one of the issues with nutritionism—the more we want to follow the nutrients and check them off, the more we rely on labels to tell us what to eat. A fresh fish fillet doesn't come with a label. Relying on ultra-processed foods, as we've seen, is antithetical to supportive emotional eating.

I remember an ad on the back of a cereal box when I was a kid that asked, "Which of these foods has more sugar?" with a photo of an apple and a photo of a bowl of Count Chocula. And then it correctly stated that an apple has more sugar, attempting—I guess—to give Count Chocula a health halo and get kids off apples. Even as a young child I knew this couldn't be right, the assertion that somehow chocolate cereal with chocolate marshmallows is a better choice than an apple. The box read: "And our bodies use the sugar in Count Chocula the same way they use the apple's sugar . . . for energy."

If you want to avoid foods that depress moods—simple sugars, refined carbs—it's best to learn to read a nutrition label. I've always been a fan of focusing on what to add and what to do rather than adhering to rules about what you can't do. We should focus on adding nutrients, according to one study in *Nutritional Review*, not on things to avoid.

A label will tell you how many of the sugars in your food are added sugars. Added sugars are usually the simple sugars that give quick bursts of energy (soon followed by the infamous sugar crash). Count Chocula's sugar is added to a product to make it highly palatable, while the apple's sugars are natural and come with the apple's fiber to slow the absorption of the sugar so your blood sugar doesn't spike. Plus we get a lot of nutrients and polyphenols from the apple that we don't get from Count Chocula. When I was a kid, labels didn't have added sugars—but they do now, and it's really helpful to check added sugars versus total sugars if you are considering an ultra-processed food.

The best thing we can do now to support our mental health, as individuals, is to adopt an eating pattern of whole foods and cooking for ourselves. People who can't cook for themselves will always be at the mercy of others' opinions of what is delicious, healthful, or worth eating— and in danger of eating only what others who can cook (or, more frequently, others who process and package food) think you should eat.

Ultra-Processed Foods

A population study of more than 140,000 people found that frequent eating of fried foods, especially fried potatoes, is associated with a 12 percent increase in risk of depression and a 7 percent increase in risk of anxiety. Humans are an ecosystem, and there are multiple reasons that someone eating more fries might have greater depression or anxiety risk, which is a big reason that causation is currently impossible to show (and usually is, with nutrition science). Do they live in an area that doesn't offer many delicious non-fried options? Are they working long hours, so they don't have energy to cook? Or are they turning to fried foods for comfort, which most of us have done at some point? The question is whether it's part of our regular eating pattern.

Bringing oil to high heat, whether for frying or for use in making non-fried ultra-processed food, produces a contaminant known as acrylamide. Acrylamide has been shown to suppress the expression of the genes that decrease the strength of the blood-brain barrier, so pathogens that naturally circulate in our blood can more easily get into the brain, potentially wreaking havoc on emotional well-being. Consumption of acrylamide is associated with neuroinflammation that is in turn associated with mental health disorders.

As Chris van Tulleken writes in 2023's *Ultra-Processed People*, "There is all the epidemiological evidence: dozens of well-conducted studies carried out independently of industry funding showing convincing links between UPF and a range of health conditions, including early death." In just the past few years, more than a dozen studies across five countries have consistently shown that consumption of ultra-processed food is associated with greater health problems—and problems happen incrementally.

To many nutrition scientists, it's not a matter of whether but of how. And mechanisms are hard to pick apart in a complex ecosystem like a human. Evidence continues to pile up that ultra-processed foods can interfere with emotional well-being and mental health. A 2023 study involving more than 31,000 women aged 42 to 62 showed that those who ate the most ultra-processed food were 50 percent likelier to develop depression than the women who ate the least amount of ultra-processed food. Fifty percent is a staggering difference. And this particular study supports stronger causation, as it used data covering a span of almost 15 years, not simply a blip in time; participants were free from depression symptoms at the beginning of the study. As is a flaw in lots of studies, most of the women were white. Most studies that are recruiting volunteers now—including the new phase of the study mentioned here, the Nurses' Health Study—prioritize diverse ethnic and racial backgrounds.

A note on choosing between sugar and artificial sweeteners for emotional well-being: if you eat sugar and are looking to decrease your sugar intake by adding artificial sweeteners, the evidence suggests you should think again. The Nurses' Health Study showed particular increases in depression and anxiety when ultra-processed food consumption included soft drinks with artificial sweeteners.

As with most dietary recommendations, it's simple but not easy. If you have the time and energy to avoid ultra-processed foods all the time, by all means do it. But ultra-processed foods exist for a reason. They are often:

» Inexpensive
» Shelf-stable, so you don't need a plan to eat them within a certain time, as with fresh food
» Delicious (science uses the term "highly palatable" because flavor is created in the brain, and ultra-processed foods are just perceived differently in the brain—we don't know why)
» Available everywhere, all the time because they can be very profitable for the sellers in a world where everyone is trying to get by—hospitals, church, schools, gas stations, etc.
» So built into the industrial infrastructure that they are increasingly the default choice for feeding a planet of 8 billion people
» Easy to eat

These are real reasons, compelling reasons, why we keep making and consuming ultra-processed food even in the face of increasing evidence that it's making our lives worse. Ultra-processed food is, simply, the easy choice in a world where there are so many other difficult choices every single day. The injustice of this is that the lower you get on the socio-economic ladder, the more basic to survival the choices often are. And when humans' survival is threatened, we usually, understandably, make the choice that will help us to survive that very minute, without looking ten years down the road.

Some nutrition scientists take the argument further, giving evidence that ultra-processed food is addictive, according to a definition of substance-use disorders (two or more symptoms of addiction in the past year, such as overconsumption and cravings, plus significant impairment and distress). A 2023 report showed that people compulsively eat foods high in refined carbohydrates and added fats, with brain effects (such as dopamine release) similar to addictive substances like nicotine and alcohol. The researchers looked at 281 studies from 36 countries.

Five Definitions of and Guidelines for Ultra-Processed Foods

Remember that this is an evolving area of science, and there is no single definition of ultra-processed foods. Some believe the lack of definition results from an effort by the ultra-processed food industry to cloud the conversation and have people spend their precious time fighting over definitions rather than creating regulations.

Definitions that try to cover literally tens of thousands of products, when we don't know their specific mechanisms, are blunt tools. That's why definitions—while absolutely necessary for regulation—can be an insidious tool that confuses us when we're just standing in the grocery store trying to choose dinner.

1. **The food is highly shelf stable but won't last more than a day or two in your house.** If a food is made to last years but you can't stop yourself from eating it in one day, it might be a food that you eat to the exclusion of other foods, decreasing the diversity of foods you eat.
2. **Be specific.** Avoid and/or—it's too vague. An ingredient list that includes "and/or" means that a company can choose to change up which ingredient is in your food, usually based on what is most available (and therefore cheapest and most profitable—your health may not be a factor).
3. **Ingredients you can buy in the grocery store.** The product should have a list of ingredients that you could buy in your regular everyday grocery store.
4. **Sugar/salt + fat = homemade.** If the food is high in both fat and sugar or salt, buy the ingredients and make it at home (second choice: buy a small-producer version of it, such as a cookie from a local bakery, which is likelier to use regular kitchen ingredients).
5. **Common sense.** There are lots of chemistry terms involved here, but the message is: use basic nutrition knowledge. I know the whole point is that we're trying to define junk, but we likely won't have unanimous agreement in our lifetimes.

The evidence is compelling enough that Colombia passed the first-ever "junk food tax" of 10 percent in 2023, rising to 15 percent in 2024 and 20 percent in 2025. The law is designed to incrementally increase the expense of junk food (intending to both decrease consumption and collect money to pay for health problems believed to be linked to ultra-processed food).

It was implemented just at the end of 2023, so no statistics are available about how it's working, although increasing taxes on products deleterious to health often have that effect.

Colombia, as well as neighboring Ecuador and Peru, already had health warning labels on ultra-processed foods with high content of added sugar and saturated fats, so there was already a working definition of which foods should be covered by the tax. Taxing an item or activity often leads to less use or participation, which is one of the philosophical purposes of a tax in the first place. But the scientific possibility of ultra-processed food addiction makes the issue more complicated—active addicts with money to spend don't always skimp on the object of their addiction. They may even look for more concentrated ways to get whatever value they get out of using. But the evidence is still preliminary, and there is a lot of debate about whether "addiction" is the correct term to apply to ultra-processed foods.

The mounting evidence is spurring talk of government regulation of ultra-processed foods. All good news, but we must remember what causes us to choose ultra-processed food in the first place, even for those of us who have access to fresh food. Alongside regulation, governments must look at ways to make fresh foods more accessible. It's more effective to say, "don't do this" when you offer an alternative.

Nutrition Studies: It's Complicated

Even with everything we know today, labs' abilities to do dietary research in humans are limited. "Nutrition is the most devilishly difficult of all the things to study in health research," says Felice Jacka, the lead author of the SMILES trial about the Mediterranean diet and mental health.

First, food research has a mechanism/causation issue. Part of this is because scientific studies are about limiting the factor you want to study and comparing it to control factors. That's the scientific method. But food is complicated, so it's hard to establish one food mechanism that causes effects in the human body. "Something we debate about in the lab is,

'What does "mechanism" even mean?'," gut microbiome researcher Peter Turnbaugh told me. His lab's members have diverse skill sets and educations to reflect the complexity of the gut microbiome.

"If I ask Ben the biochemist, he has a very different view of what he thinks a mechanism is than I may," Turnbaugh says. In our conversation about mechanisms, Turnbaugh warned me against what he calls "diet nihilism." In science sometimes, the more you know, the more you realize you don't know. And not knowing everything doesn't mean we should just throw our hands up and eat chips all day.

Second, it's difficult to get people to report accurately what they eat and how much of it.

A study published in 2021 showed that research subjects who were told to record everything they ate consistently underreported the amount of calories they ate each day. The study reported "substantial" underestimation of calories consumed to the point that the study warned that underestimations should be considered when analyzing self-reported data. The underestimation applied to all kinds of memory-based recall—food frequency questionnaires (do you eat these foods often-sometimes-never), recording everything you eat based on a 24-hour recall, and estimating food records are the most commonly used for research. Dani Reed, a researcher at Monell, told me, "Short of putting a webcam on the top of someone's head, looking down to see what goes in the mouth, it's very hard to get super accurate measures. It's as good as the person doing the recording and the person doing the interviewing."

If you had to record your eating habits, would you record licking a bit of brownie batter off a spoon? In the scientific method, the lick matters.

Plus, if someone recalls that they ate two slices of bread at a restaurant, there is no telling what the ingredients are. Even if someone says they ate a carrot, there can be differences in nutrient density between a carrot recently pulled from the ground that you bought at the farmers' market and one that's been kicking around a bodega for a month. And each body processes food differently, depending on a lot of the factors we've talked about, including your particular gut bacteria.

Third, as we've seen, some studies can't be performed with humans for multiple reasons. Conventional medical ethics prohibit some stud-ies in humans that can be done in animals, such as what happens when you cut the vagus nerve in a mouse. You can't cut the vagus nerve of a human for research, according to current medical ethics. Plus sometimes labs don't have enough money to do human studies—it's often way more complicated and expensive to study humans than rodents, and there isn't enough research money available for people to do all the kinds of studies they want.

The NIH study that tracked consumption of ultra-processed food and weight gain was really expensive. They housed 40 people on the NIH cam-pus for four weeks. Researchers put participants in metabolic chambers for hours to see how many calories they burned. And that doesn't even account for the screening of hundreds of people to see who can be a par-ticipant before the study even starts.

You can't lock people up and control what they eat for long periods of time unless you have a lot of space and a lot of money and people will-ing to be locked up for some period of time and have every bite they take controlled and measured and watched and their bodily fluids tested. That's one reason why many food studies are based on dietary recall. Also it's a reason why some food intake studies seem small. Only 40 people? Only four weeks? Yes, because getting more people to do that for longer periods of time can be difficult. Food is intensely personal and intimate, and shar-ing that information can be a deal-breaker for some.

Fourth, for food studies, it's hard to blind people to what they eat. (There are some ways around this, such as feeding equal-looking dishes of yogurt with very different levels of probiotics.) If they're eating ham-burgers instead of salmon, it's easy to guess which control group they're in. "It's very difficult to do the very tight type of science that researchers like where you control everything and measure everything. But you've got to start. And in nutrition science, you have to look at the totality of the evidence," says Jacka.

Science requires exact measurements. A trio of British studies of wild blueberries—which was not funded by any industry—showed the fruit's effect on mood. They randomized and controlled the studies by turning the blueberries into a powder and that powder into a drink. Two studies examined the short-term effect of blueberries on mood (two hours after ingestion), and the other examined the long-term effect (four weeks after daily drinks) in people without mental health disorders. All three studies showed positive effects on mood, ranging from small to medium.

Food Prescriptions

When we talked about blood sugar, we looked at a recent finding that people with diabetes who are food insecure experience low blood sugar episodes two times more frequently than those who are not food insecure. Extreme low blood sugar, or hypoglycemia, can be deadly.

Recently, insurance companies and food-related companies, such as grocery stores, are seeing the potential financial benefit of subsidizing customers' produce as a way of saving money in the future. Programs known as "food prescriptions" can vary widely, from lowering the cost of fruits and vegetables to full-blown cooking classes and complete meal delivery for people with chronic conditions. These programs try to address the frightening statistic that currently only one in ten Americans eats the daily recommended amount of fruits and vegetables.

Some recent developments that show the exploding interest in produce prescriptions, from private industry to government programs, include:

» The grocery store Kroger has partnered with the meal-preparation company Performance Kitchen to provide medically tailored meals for people with diet-related conditions.

» To address the lack of nutrition education in medical schools—71 percent do not reach the minimum benchmark of twenty-five hours of nutrition education recommended by the National Academy of Sciences—some schools are creating culinary medicine centers. The goal of these centers is to provide basic food knowledge for medical students to pass on to their patients.

» Instacart, the grocery delivery service, and Kaiser Permanente have a pilot program with medically tailored nutrition advice and a grocery produce stipend (read: free food) for people with diet-related conditions. Participants will have key diet-quality indicators measured during the program, such as blood sugar. It's one of several programs Instacart is investing in with other companies as part of its health initiative announced in 2022. These programs are potentially good for Instacart's bottom line and good for people who need both better nutrition and better access to nutrition—grocery delivery ensures fruit and vegetable access. Some studies show that online grocery shopping leads to lower diversity in diet (likely from just clicking "buy again"), so produce vouchers may encourage shoppers to try new things. Online grocery shopping has benefits too: people tend to purchase fewer impulse buys, such as candy, which is usually at the checkout counter at a brick-and-mortar store.

» A 2023 study looked at effects of a twenty-four-week produce delivery program for people in rural areas who have type 2 diabetes. Participants had a significant reduction in A1C, a measure of a person's blood sugar over a period of several months.

» Food literacy programs are on the rise internationally, with the goal of giving people the knowledge and skills to select, prepare, and eat fruits and vegetables. One Australian study found that after people were educated with a food literacy program, participants had a significant improvement in number of vegetables eaten.

» Mindful eating programs are becoming more common to address the "how" of eating, not just the "what." By bringing attention to the eating experience, one study showed that participants with high blood pressure adhered more closely to a diet to decrease hypertension (the DASH diet) over eight weeks.

» A Chicago hospital distributes free fruits and vegetables to food-insecure patients and patients with food-related conditions, such as diabetes. Some of the produce comes from another hospital outside the city, which transformed two acres of its campus into a "farmacy" growing 100 varieties of produce for the Food Is Medicine program.

» Giant Food grocery stores employ six nutritionists, described as "concierges for healthy eating," to travel to 165 regional stores to teach food-is-medicine programs. The company partners with local organizations, such as nonprofits or physicians' offices, to give fruit and vegetable prescriptions—financial incentives—linked to the chain's loyalty cards. Customers are more likely to use the benefits when they are linked to standard loyalty cards, rather than a separate voucher that cashiers must be trained to use.

"Food is medicine" is the phrase currently used to describe initiatives like these. I'm not looking to create infighting among we who are trying to promote the science behind the power of eating, but I don't know if that label is particularly helpful for individual eaters. It bifurcates food into "medical" food and "nonmedical" food, which sounds dangerously close to "good" food and "bad" food. It doesn't factor in the cultural importance of food; food can have the same effects as drugs, but it's so much more (I know, this would be a terrible slogan). I get that we need to medicalize food to get insurance companies involved in food reimbursement, so it's a great industry message but maybe not the best message for an individual deciding what to buy when faced with aisles of easy, inexpensive, ready-to-eat ultra-processed food in the grocery store.

Insurance companies are businesses, so they need to see that the bottom-line financial benefit from reimbursing for food is in their favor. But "food is medicine" is historically not the most compelling message for people choosing food on an everyday basis (in part for pleasure). Messages are all around us about how food can improve physical health. By focusing on emotional well-being, we are balancing the immediate well-being that delicious food brings us with the long-term effects of our food choices. It's not the lack of information; it's the lack of actual on-the-ground food choices, and private industry subsidizing fruits and vegetables may go a long way to making the long-term emotional well-being choices the easiest choices to make.

There is evidence that people perceive foods that have health halos— the perception that it is a good choice for health—as less delicious than other foods. One study showed that healthiness and deliciousness were inversely related. The less that food is introduced to eaters as "healthy," the more delicious participants rated the food both during and after eating it.

Researching health effects of diet is hard. Some reactions can be studied and measured and some can't—the pleasure of biting into a warm cake with a melty center or the satisfying snap of a snow pea between our teeth. Additionally, as we know from both science and experience, mental health and emotional well-being are complex and dependent on many factors.

And even when we do have more information, it takes time for the government to move and act and reroute funding. We had a ton of research that lung cancer and smoking were associated, but it wasn't until 1969 that labels were put on cigarette packs, warning that smoking causes cancer, and it wasn't until the late 1980s that we started banning smoking in the enclosed space of airplanes. My high school in Connecticut in the 1990s still had a smoking lounge for students. It takes a while for science to turn into policy. This is good because if we didn't have a process, every kooky idea would have the same weight. It can be not as beneficial, though, when there is groundbreaking, peer-reviewed research that can help people. In the meantime, we can act as our own advocates by eating to support our mental health.

It's great to want to protect our minds in old age. It's also great to enjoy our time getting to old age. Brains are not just there to produce, produce, produce more work for your job. Or, as life coach Martha Beck told me in 2020, "Your body is more than a way to get your brain from meeting to meeting."

In the next recipe, you'll make your own salad dressing, which is an easy way to start caring for your brain health. Many bottled salad dressings are made with industrially produced seed oils (they are generally less expensive than olive oil), which—as part of a regular eating pattern—may negatively affect brain health.

Three Emotional Well-Being Add-Ons for Your Meal

1. **Microgreens (aka vegetable confetti).** When you see a package of microgreens in your grocery store's produce section, it's easy to pass up as some kind of nonsense, but microgreens are densely packed with many emotional well-being nutrients. You can easily grow them at home, too, as they're simply very young plants with a couple of tiny leaves (if left unpicked, a broccoli microgreen would turn into a whole broccoli stalk).
2. **Chopped nuts.** Nut consumption in itself is associated with lower risk of depression. And when added to simple sugars, nuts may slow down your blood sugar spike by adding protein, fats, and fiber to the meal.
3. **Menu creativity.** One of the huge benefits of cooking: you make it, you get to name it. A dish's name may help your brain get more pleasure out of your food. "Hannah's Crunchy Fresh Nantucket Cod" sounds more delicious than "fish sticks."

Pizza Salad

The food in Los Angeles is terrific. The gorgeous weather allows Ange-lenos to grow produce year-round, so something delicious is always in season. This recipe is based on a simple salad from La Scala, an Italian restaurant in Beverly Hills founded by actor James Dean and restau-rateur Jean Leon (and still owned by the same family). It is a terrific example of how meat can be used in small amounts for big flavor, a characteristic of the Mediterranean diet. Although science shows that cured meats should not be part of a regular eating pattern for mental health, this recipe uses uncured pepperoni sparingly, alongside lots of vegetables and beans. Big, punchy flavors, lots of fiber, tons of pleasure.

Iceberg lettuce adds crunchy texture and lasts longer in your fridge than some other greens. The beans marinate in the dressing, so the salad stands up well in the refrigerator for several hours—and the marinade helps soften often-tough kale leaves too. I've made this salad in a mason jar with the beans marinating on the bottom and layers of salad on top. When I'm hungry, I just pull out a jar of homemade salad.

This recipe has one of my favorite food hacks: making salad dress-ing in an almost-empty mustard jar. Leftover mustard clinging to the sides of the jar flavors the dressing. The topped jar makes a perfect vessel for shaking to combine, it's one less dish to wash, and there's no whisk needed. You can store dressing right in the jar until you're ready to use it. One other reason to make your own dressing: Many bottled salad dressings are made with industrially produced seed oils (they are generally less expensive than olive oil), which—as part of a regular eating pattern—may negatively affect brain health.

SERVES 4

⅓ cup extra-virgin olive oil

3 tablespoons red wine vinegar

2 teaspoons Dijon mustard

1 tablespoon grated pecorino Romano cheese

½ teaspoon kosher salt

½ teaspoon freshly ground black pepper

1 (15.5-ounce) can cannellini beans, drained

2 cups stemmed and chopped kale leaves

1 head iceberg lettuce, core removed and leaves chopped into
  bite-sized pieces

2 ounces uncured pepperoni slices, cut into ribbons (optional)

2 ounces shredded mozzarella cheese

¼ cup sun-dried tomatoes

In an empty mustard jar, add the oil, vinegar, mustard, pecorino, and salt and pepper, and shake until combined. Whatever mustard is on the sides of the jar will dissolved into the dressing. If you don't have a jar available, whisk these ingredients in a bowl until combined.

In a medium bowl, toss the beans and kale together with the dressing.

To the bowl, add the lettuce on top of the beans. Sprinkle the pepperoni, mozzarella, and sun-dried tomatoes on top of the lettuce. At this point you can toss the salad and serve. Or you can store the bowl in the fridge for up to several hours, toss, and then serve. If you're transporting it somewhere, leave the salad untossed until before serving.

CHAPTER 6

How to Eat for Emotional Well-Being

"When engaged in eating, the brain should be the servant of the stomach."
—AGATHA CHRISTIE

A S YOU KNOW BY NOW, food is a critical component of emotional well-being. But research shows that focusing on rigidity and perfection can compromise the exact emotional wellness that we are pursuing. A big part of mental health is flexibility, bending to respond to life's events that you have no power over (along with working on the areas where you do have power). That's why it's critical to focus on manageable, achievable goals that ultimately change our eating patterns.

And being able to identify and work on the ways we try to justify poor eating patterns is especially critical so our goals are based in the reality of who we are. Unwanted habits and patterns always have a reason behind them. The goal is to figure out the reason and find a new way to live that is more in line with our priorities.

Food writers sometimes get asked what our "point of view" or "food philosophy" is. My food philosophy is that my grandparents would have thought it was hysterical to have a food philosophy. For most of history, most of humanity cooked whatever they had. There is still no room for perfection in a home kitchen; your kitchen is crowded enough. Striving to be perfect will cause unhappiness or lack of confidence or—tragically and worst of all—abandoning cooking altogether. It's the cooking version of orthorexia, an obsession with clean and pure foods. It's OK not to be a professional chef. You are good at so many other things. When I choose foods these days—which recipe to cook or what to order on a menu or what to buy when I'm hungry at a CVS—I think of the acronym PING: pleasure, inflammation, nutrients, gut microbiome. Ideally, my meal choices serve at least two of these ways to eat for mental health. Sometimes we all eat just for pleasure, but PING reminds me of my commitment to a better eating pattern. I use this acronym all the time, and it has helped me distill the science and reframe how I make food choices.

The following specific recommendations combine peer-reviewed science from several fields about how food affects emotional well-being. They follow the four elements to pay attention to when eating for emotional wellness: the microbiome, inflammation, nutrients, and pleasure. These are distinct concepts that influence and intersect with each other because the human body is a system and emotions are complicated. Furthermore, when you're getting started, focusing on one part of eating for emotional wellness at a time—for example, focusing on eating for your microbiome—one week at a time is a cycle that is both familiar and constantly changing.

Each week you'll focus on a different part of supporting mental and emotional wellness. Rotating focus every week is both manageable and reinforcing. It gives variety not just to your overall eating pattern but for your brain.

Eating to support emotional well-being allows for all kinds of dietary restrictions or other advice from your physician about your specific body. You can use the already existing billions of recipes—you don't have to toss beloved cookbooks or swear off your favorite recipe websites. And each week supports the other weeks—some foods that support a diverse microbiome will also guard against inflammation. And it helps look at food in a sane, sustainable, and science-supported way: You don't get so caught up in nutrients that you forget about pleasure. You don't get so caught up in pleasure that you forget about inflammation.

Eating for emotional wellness is flexible and will fit in with most other eating plans that you may want to try or have already figured out work for you. This is a dietary pattern that can fit into most lifestyles and is focused on adding beneficial foods rather than restriction. The dissonance between what you know you "should" eat and what you're actually eating can itself create difficult emotions—this plan allows you to make incremental, easy, and delicious changes.

And, because eating for emotional wellness is a process, each week can build on the previous without boredom. We've seen that the average American gets almost 60 percent of calories from ultra-processed foods—you may be on the high or low side of that average, but if you eat any ultra-processed food at all, you have a reason for it. It can be difficult to go from the convenience and/or pleasure bombs that ultra-processed foods provide to spending time sourcing and cooking ingredients that will give lots of pleasure. We may not be able to do it all in one month. And that's OK because our senses are, well, sensitive; subtle changes can make a big difference.

It's tough, I know! When you're in the middle of intense emotions, self-care can go by the wayside. I've had times in my life when I was leaking tears and hemorrhaging money, and that's an awful feeling. And when you're not looking forward to the future, it's hard to say to yourself, *I'll make better food choices so I can feel better in the future.* That's why it's such great news that the changes can be gradual, to develop into an eating pattern.

There are three recommendations for each week, and I've included a personal favorite recipe, food hack, or DIY project for that week. You can choose to focus on one per day at first, and as you repeat the cycle and familiarize yourself with mental-health-supporting foods, you can challenge yourself to incorporate all the recommendations at once. This is how you can turn these steps into a new dietary pattern.

The small changes of the four-week focus plan become part of your eating pattern. After focusing on eating for emotional well-being, your eating pattern will ideally include:

» At least 5 cups of produce (heavy on the vegetables, particularly leafy greens) every day;

» Fermented food every day;

» Seafood two to three times per week;

» Whole grains (whenever you choose to eat grains);

» Beans and legumes, such as lentils;

» Nuts;

» Healthful fat like olive oil;

» Cooking, preparing, or choosing ingredients/growing your food at least once per day; and

» Eating with another person at least once per day (eating at your desk while other people walk by doesn't count).

That may be very different from how you eat now; you may want to use the four-week plan more than once to get yourself back on the track of eating for emotional health or when you are in a particularly emotionally difficult time. Remember, no change is small! Here are some specific recommendations based on the research and my conversations with scientists.

WEEK ONE
Microbiome

**For the first week, focus on science-backed
ways of improving the diversity and species
of bacteria in your gut microbiome.**

PROBIOTICS

Eat at least one fermented food each day. Check the label for two things:
First, that it has no added sugar (it can be harmful to good bacteria).
Fermented products have natural sugars, so it's OK for the label to list
something under "total sugars"—but under "added sugars" it should
say 0. Second, be sure that it contains live, active bacteria. Products that
are pasteurized after fermenting will not retain as many or any of the
beneficial bacteria. Do not heat fermented foods; heat will destroy a lot
of beneficial bacteria. Good fermented food choices include:

» Kombucha with no added sugar.
» Fermented vegetables. Remember that fermentation is a subset of pickling; not all pickles are fermented. Fermented vegetables (including "pickles") will likely be in the refrigerator
   section and will not list vinegar as an ingredient. Look for
   kimchi, Korean fermented and spiced mixed vegetables.
» Fermented cottage cheese. Most commercial cottage cheese is
   not fermented, but you can find fermented cottage cheese by
   looking at the label.
» Yogurt. Try buying plain and adding your own fresh fruit
   and/or honey. If you buy a pre-flavored yogurt, look for as few
   added sugars or artificial sweeteners as possible.
» Kefir. This comes in a bottle and is sometimes known as
   "drinkable yogurt." As with yogurt, make sure there are as

few added sugars as possible. If this is your first time drinking kefir, try a few kinds—they vary widely in taste.

» Miso paste. Miso is a seasoning made from fermented soy-beans or barley.

PREBIOTICS

Eat at least 25 grams of fiber each day for women, 38 for men. To level up, pay specific attention to soluble fiber, which is what your good microbes thrive on. Some great sources of soluble fiber include garlic, onions, oats, apples, bananas, black and kidney beans, avocado, and broccoli.

DIVERSITY

Buy and eat 30 different plants in one week, and make sure they are as unprocessed as possible. (The studies looked at different species of plants, so different types of apples or kale count as the same. But if you're trying to keep track of how many different kinds of kale you're eating, you're probably doing better than you think.) Thirty plants may seem daunting, but remember that you're probably already a third of the way there: wheat, corn, rice, lettuce, tomato, onion, and bananas all count. Go to the grocery store with the goal of increasing your plant variety and total consumption. When I'm focusing on diversity, I'll actually count how many different plants are in my cart to make sure I'm on track. And I allow for extra time in the checkout line because it takes some time to ring up one apple, one banana, one kiwifruit, one papaya, etc.

Homemade Fermented Vegetables

Sauerkraut is easy, has two ingredients, and massaging cabbage is meditative. You can do it when you're watching TV or on a work call—also great for kids you want to keep busy.

MAKES ONE 2-QUART JAR

1 whole green cabbage (about 2 pounds)
1 tablespoon kosher salt

Remove the wilted outer leaves of the cabbage; save one and discard the rest. Cut the cabbage into quarters; remove and discard the core. Slice the cabbage into ribbons.

Place the cabbage ribbons in a bowl and add the kosher salt. Massage the cabbage for about 5 to 10 minutes, until the cabbage releases some of its liquid (5 minutes is sufficient, but you may really enjoy it, so feel free to do it for 10 minutes).

Put the cabbage and its released liquid into a 2-quart mason jar, poking the cabbage down to make sure it's covered in its own liquid. Place the reserved wilted cabbage leaf on top of the ribbons, then place a clean cloth over the jar opening and fasten the cloth with a rubber band. If the cabbage is ever poking out above the water, add just enough water to cover the cabbage.

Otherwise, leave it alone for 3 to 10 days—you'll see bubbles on the surface showing that bacteria are active, feeding on the sugar that naturally occurs in vegetables. Start tasting the cabbage after 3 days. When it tastes right to you, remove the cloth, put a top on the jar, and store in the refrigerator for up to a month. The longer it sits, the tangier it gets.

NOTE: If you don't care for cabbage, you can ferment pretty much any vegetable, but some are more crowd-pleasing than others.

continued

Vegetables that ferment well include carrots, cauliflower, sliced cucumber, radishes, green beans—even garlic cloves, each clove separated from the head and peeled. Just put the cleaned, cut vegetables in a mason jar and pour in a mixture of 1 tablespoon kosher salt dissolved in 2 cups of water. Make sure the vegetables are covered with liquid and let the jar sit for a week or two. When the vegetables taste good to you, put a top on the jar and store in the refrigerator for up to a month.

———

WEEK TWO
Inflammation

This week focuses on anti-inflammatory foods, which can reduce the possibility of inflammatory markers, like the protein cytokine, potentially affecting brain function.

Inflammatory markers can come from the biological effects of stress; food preparation is a great way to use the energy your body produces when you're stressed but you're not using (because there's no actual tiger to run away from). You can activate your parasympathetic nervous system (known as our rest-and-digest nervous system) by doing relaxing things that allow you to breathe deeply.

FOCUS ON PANTRY-FRIENDLY ANTI-INFLAMMATORY FOODS

Beans or legumes, tomatoes, nuts, olive oil, leafy greens, fatty fish (sounds like ingredients for an amazing salad, to be honest). Spices can be anti-inflammatory; turmeric is a spice of particular interest recently because it (along with oregano) has the highest level of antioxidants. Turmeric's active ingredient is curcumin, which, in a meta-analysis, was protective of the brain and effective in reducing symptoms of depression. Keep tea in your pantry too; black tea can help reduce cortisol levels, and green tea has an amino acid that helps with dopamine production.

MINDFUL FOOD PREPARATION

Try some repetitive, easy cooking techniques, such as:

> » Kneading. "Breaditation" is the meditative act of making bread—the repetitive kneading and folding can shift our brains in a relaxed, mindful state. Notice the changes to the

dough, how it goes from tender to stretchy and bumpy to silky—if you make bread regularly, you'll eventually learn what the feeling of the dough says about how the bread will turn out, but that won't all happen in one day. It's a process toward a pattern, which is a great life lesson. Next time you have a day off, try making some bread without rushing and see how it feels. If you're more time-pressed, buying ready-made pizza dough and turning it into pizza crust is a fantastic start.

» Grinding. Try crushing whole black peppercorns with a mortar and pestle instead of buying pre-ground pepper.

» Smashing. Try smashing garlic cloves with a blunt object to remove the paper skin, or tenderizing meat. Physical activity can support your body by using up the bursts of cortisol and adrenaline and increased heart rate that can come with intense emotions.

» Picking. Picking leaves off herb stems can be maddening when you're rushed for time but meditative when you give yourself time to do it. Fresh herbs, we know, can improve taste perception, so it's always nice to have a bowl of, say, parsley to toss over otherwise humdrum eggs or even a box of takeout or a frozen pizza. My favorite is thyme—I pick thyme leaves off stems while I watch videos; the smell is amazing.

STEADY YOUR BLOOD SUGAR

The biological effects of intense emotions like anger or fear can send blood sugar soaring and dropping when your body releases stored glucose, and from emotionally unsupportive food choices. One study looked at 107 married couples over three weeks. The couples were instructed to stick between zero and fifty-one needles into a doll representing their spouse each night, depending on how aggressive they felt. The lower their blood sugar at night, the more pins they stuck in the spouse doll. Anti-inflammatory foods—whole grains, nuts, vegetables, cinnamon—are usually also good for steady blood sugar. And don't skip meals or drink alcohol on an empty stomach, both of which can cause dips in blood sugar.

Roasted Ratatouille

Ratatouille is often made as a stew, throwing a bunch of summer vegetables into one pot and letting them all mix and melt together. Roasted ratatouille is a leveled-up memory food—I like the flavors in the traditional dish but not the consistency—made way better with just a shift in technique. Roasting is a typical French method of making ratatouille, and to me it's night-and-day different from the stew. Roasting allows each vegetable to keep some of its own shape, definition, and flavor, so this ratatouille is a mélange of distinct flavors and textures. It makes a great side dish for fish, chicken, meat, or eggs—it's also fantastic on its own, or:

- » On grilled bread as an appetizer, topped with chive blossoms from my backyard when I'm feeling fancy;
- » Pureed for a few seconds in a blender, without cheese, for an incredibly complex pasta sauce or vegetable jam
- » Mixed with a little Greek yogurt and lemon juice to make a dip for pita chips; and
- » Smushed onto a piece of toast and topped with a poached egg. Getting vegetables in at breakfast can create a virtuous cycle, like exercising in the morning.

You can do a lot with this one dish, and your home will smell like a rustic old French farmhouse. This is prep-heavy, with all the vegetable chopping, but worth it, even in the winter, when vegetables may not be so great where you live (roasting concentrates flavors so a subpar tomato turns caramelly). And there is no more delicious way to get a ton of fiber in one shot.

I used to make this without bell peppers because my then significant other didn't eat them. One of the best parts of reclaiming

continued

*your life after you've lost yourself in a relationship is eating the things
you gave up because it was too inconvenient to make two versions.*

MAKES SIX I-CUP SERVINGS

1 pint cherry tomatoes (preferably multicolored), halved
2 medium zucchini (about 1¼ pounds), cut into ½-inch cubes
1 medium red onion (about ½ pound), sliced into thin half-moons
1 medium eggplant (about 1¼ pounds), skin on, cut into 1-inch cubes
1 bell pepper (red, orange, or yellow), seeded, stemmed, and sliced
    into ¼-inch strips
5 garlic cloves, peeled and smashed into pieces with the side of a
    knife or minced
1 tablespoon fresh thyme leaves
⅓ cup extra-virgin olive oil
1 teaspoon kosher salt
½ teaspoon ground black pepper
½ cup fresh basil leaves, sliced into ribbons (divided)
Grated Parmesan cheese, for topping (optional)

Heat the oven to 425°F. In a large bowl, toss together the tomatoes, zucchini, onion, eggplant, bell pepper, garlic, and thyme.
Drizzle the olive oil over the vegetables, then sprinkle the salt and
pepper and toss everything together until evenly coated. Arrange
the vegetables evenly in a single layer on two 13-by-18-inch sheet
pans. Place the pans on separate oven racks. Roast until the vegetables are tender and browned, 45 to 60 minutes, switching the
pans on the racks halfway through. Remove the pans from the
oven and cool slightly. Place the vegetables in a large serving bowl
and toss with ⅓ cup of basil, then top with the remaining basil
and cheese (if using).

NOTE: Can be made 2 days in advance and stored in an airtight
container in the refrigerator. Great cold or hot. Freeze in airtight
container for up to 2 months.

WEEK THREE
Nutrients

Certain nutrients can be depleted by the biological
processes that accompany emotions. This week focus on
nutrient-dense foods that have emotional-well-being-
supporting properties. In addition to recommendations,
I've included a list of some nutrients that have been
studied for brain-protective properties. You can try
them out, depending on your specific needs.

DHA/EPA

Eat seafood three times per week, particularly fatty cold-water fish—they
tend to be highest in DHA and EPA. If you already do that, you can focus
on specific types of fish: oysters, tuna, salmon (canned is fine), anchovies,
sardines, and mackerel. If you buy canned tuna, the kind that is highest in
DHA and EPA is usually white albacore packed in water.

FLAVONOIDS

We're going to get the whole color wheel on our plates this week. Get a
5-cup clear container and fill it with mostly vegetables and some fruit in
the morning. You should be able to see multiple colors from the outside so
you can ensure a spectrum of flavonoids.

RED: radicchio, strawberries, cranberries
GREEN: broccoli, peas, green beans
ORANGE: carrots, butternut squash, papayas
YELLOW: yellow peppers, yellow tomatoes, pears
BLUE/PURPLE: eggplant, blueberries, grapes

Be sure to eat one green leafy vegetable every day (the darker the better) and include one you didn't have last month. Examples include spinach, arugula, watercress, kale, collard greens, and beet greens. Eating microgreens, tiny leafy seedlings, is a handy secret too. They can have up to 10 times (or more) nutritional value than a fully grown plant.

IF YOU EAT ANIMAL PRODUCTS, RAISE THE QUALITY

Try grass-fed beef or organic chicken. Grass-fed beef, for example, has some omega-3 fatty acids, whereas grain-fed beef has little or none.

Emotional Wellness Nutrients

B Vitamins

THIAMINE (AKA B$_1$): Fish, whole grains, meat. Thiamine can help relieve symptoms of anxiety disorders, fatigue, and depression. Thiamine protects the hippocampus and improves the body's ability to handle stress.

VITAMIN B$_6$: Poultry, peanuts, oats, bananas. Vitamin B$_6$ is a precursor to creating mood-stabilizing neurotransmitters, such as serotonin, and it supports the nervous system generally, but we need to replace B$_6$ every day. B$_6$ is associated with improved regulation of anxiety, depression, and irritability.

VITAMIN B$_9$ (AKA FOLATE, FOLIC ACID): Legumes (beans, peas, lentils), black-eyed peas, brussels sprouts, romaine lettuce, avocado, asparagus, leafy greens, beets, citrus fruits, green peas, kidney beans. Levels of folic acid are much lower in people with depression than in people without; the higher your folate level, the lower your risk of depression. Low levels of folic acid are linked to loss of brain cells (particularly in the hippocampus), which in turn increases the risk of depression. Low folate is linked to poor response to antidepressant medication.

VITAMIN B$_{12}$: Eggs, meat, poultry, fish, milk, oysters. Lack of B$_{12}$ is linked to poor response to antidepressant medication.

Magnesium

Avocado, dark chocolate, nuts (almonds, cashews, Brazil nuts), beans (black), pumpkin seeds, whole grains, fatty fish (salmon, mackerel, halibut), leafy greens, spices. Magnesium helps with sleep and can lower stress levels. Low levels of magnesium are associated with anxiety, and more magnesium can have a stabilizing effect on anxiety symptoms. In one study, students taking a test had increased levels of magnesium in their urine, so we need to replace the magnesium our body uses or secretes when it's stressed.

Potassium

Bananas, spices, white beans, sweet potato, avocado, spinach, salmon. In one study, people with depression experienced an improved mood when they ate more potassium. Low levels of potassium are linked to mental fatigue and moodiness. In another study, children who ate a combination of both high-sodium and low-potassium foods had increased depressive symptoms. It is estimated that 20 percent of people with mental disorders have potassium deficiency.

Selenium

Whole grains, Brazil nuts. Low selenium is linked to depressed mood; high levels of selenium are linked to higher mood. Selenium protects against human cell oxidation, which can lead to inflammation. Selenium modulates neurotransmitter production systems, including for dopamine, serotonin, and noradrenaline.

Vitamin A

Liver, eggs, fish, milk, sweet potatoes, black-eyed peas, carrots, spinach. Vitamin A supports the adrenal glands, which help to reduce stress and anxiety. In the body, vitamin A turns into retinoic acid, which promotes production of neurotransmitters. Vitamin A deficiency has been linked with shrinking of the hippocampus.

Vitamin C

Citrus fruit, kiwifruit, peppers, cruciferous vegetables. Vitamin C may play a role in reducing cortisol, increasing dopamine production, reducing inflammation, and supporting treatment of stress-related disorders. Vitamin C deficiency is linked to fatigue and depression. The adrenal gland is one of the organs with the highest concentration of vitamin C. Tests showed that the body releases vitamin C in response to the stress hormones that regulate the fight-or-flight hormone cortisol. When stress hormones are present, vitamin C is released from the adrenal gland. As discussed earlier, humans are one of the few mammals who can't make their own vitamin C.

Zinc
Oysters, beans, nuts, pumpkin seeds, beef, liver, egg yolks. Zinc levels may be lower in people with depression and anxiety, and zinc deficiency is linked with emotional instability, irritability, and deficits in social behavior. Zinc reduces brain inflammation and may help antidepressants work more effectively. The hippocampus has high levels of zinc, so this mineral helps the nervous system function, particularly the vagus nerve. Zinc supports production of serotonin, dopamine, and conversion of short-chain fatty acids (ALA) into long-chain fatty acids (DHA, EPA).

Iron
Spices (cumin, turmeric, thyme), meat. Iron is required for our bodies to produce dopamine and serotonin. Low dopamine is linked to fatigue, anxiety, depression, and poor concentration. Iron deficiency is linked with anxiety and depression. Iron also protects neurons.

Vitamin D
Oily fish, any product that is fortified with vitamin D, such as dairy, eggs. Vitamin D is linked to the expression of 10,000 genes that regulate mood and emotion, including genes that make serotonin and oxytocin. People with depression and anxiety often have lower levels of vitamin D. Low vitamin D is linked to seasonal affective disorder, depression, and panic disorder. Vitamin D is able to cross the blood-brain barrier to get to neurons, decreasing inflammation.

Hummus

Once I helped a hummus brand open a pop-up restaurant in Georgetown. I spent days at the world's largest hummus factory, developing recipes and eating the creamy dip by the spoonful. We incorporated it into salad dressing, used it as a tasty soup thickener, ate it as a base for fried eggs, and spread it on sandwiches. At the end of every day, I was surprised by how calm I felt after long and hectic days away from home.

It turns out, hummus is full of vitamin B_6 and a deficiency of B_6 is linked to depression. It also has magnesium to support sleep, a frequent casualty of anger. Tahini, an essential ingredient for hummus, is just ground toasted sesame seeds. It contains antioxidants called lignans to protect against free radical damage and inflammation. Good fats like tahini and olive oil also lower blood pressure, which can soar when we live in fear. As I incorporated hummus into my eating pattern, I experienced pronounced effects. Every body is different, and we know there is no single food that can claim "eat me and you'll feel better." But try it out—eating hummus with vegetables combines two powerful, potentially emotionally supportive foods.

When the pop-up opened, we had a hummus topping party. I put out dozens of different toppings—all of which work terrifically well with hummus. Some of my favorites (that are also supportive of mental health):

» Pickled ginger
» Chopped fermented vegetables, such as cucumber
» Preserved lemon
» Kimchi
» Chopped nuts (hazelnuts, pistachios)
» Mango chutney
» Salsa verde
» Mint chutney
» Spices (za'atar, harissa powder)
» Fresh chopped herbs (dill, cilantro, oregano)

continued

MAKES 1¾ CUPS

4 tablespoons lemon juice (approximately 1 juicy lemon)
¼ cup tahini, well stirred
1 tablespoon aquafaba (liquid from the can of chickpeas)
1 to 2 garlic cloves, minced
¼ cup extra-virgin olive oil
1 (15½-ounce) can chickpeas, drained (some liquid reserved)
½ teaspoon kosher salt
1 to 3 tablespoons hot water

In a food processor, combine the lemon juice, tahini, and aqua-faba. Process for about 1 minute, until the mixture looks fluffy. With the motor running, add the garlic and oil and process for a few seconds. Stop the motor and add the chickpeas and salt. Process for about 1 minute, stopping to scrape the sides of the bowl if necessary, until the hummus is the consistency you want. (Sometimes I like it a little chunkier, sometimes very smooth. You get to decide. It's your hummus.) The hummus might be very thick. If so, add the hot water, a tablespoon at a time, and pulse until the water is incorporated and the hummus is how you like it. If you have a mortar and pestle lying around the kitchen, try using them instead of a food processor.

———

WEEK FOUR
Pleasure

This week, focus on your food pleasure without
relying on long-term health-damaging processed
foods. Focusing on pleasure means looking at ways
to heighten our food pleasure. Some options:

CREATE NEW FOOD MEMORIES

We create new food memories every day, and we teach ourselves how to
eat every day. Food is one of the best ways to evoke memories because
eating saturates the five senses. Connecting good food with happy memories helps us associate those foods with happiness. Creating our own food
memories means making sure we eat particularly well when we are feeling
good—that's our window of opportunity to create happy associations with
food that will help our long-term wellness. For example, at a restaurant,
choose something from the menu that is different from your usual but still
looks delicious—and will satisfy your goals of supporting your microbiome, fulfilling your nutrient needs, or decreasing inflammation. We can
create our own new comfort foods by associating health-supporting foods
with good times.

HAVE SOMEONE OVER FOR FOOD YOU'VE COOKED

And don't make a big production out of it. If you're overwhelmed by the
idea of cooking, decide on making one simple recipe really well—soup or
spaghetti and meatballs. Or try drizzling homemade infused oil over your
takeout—if you can put oil in a pot, you can make infused oil. Cooking
offers a sense of accomplishment from creating something, and the repeti-
tion and familiarity of serving one dish will make it less stressful. Remind
yourself: This isn't about perfection, it's about community. Plus the smell
of something delicious on your own stove is irresistible.

EXPERIMENT WITH NEW FOOD PLEASURES

Experiment with one new evidence-backed way to heighten food pleasure:

» Go to a new farmers' market or a specialized food store or counter, such as a butcher. If you have questions about what you're buying, ask—they may have answers. It doesn't have to be fancy.

» Experiment with plates of different colors, shapes, and sizes to see if they affect how your brain perceives the food's flavor. Do the same with cutlery of different weights, shapes, and sizes. Pay attention to things like how many tines the fork has, or how long they are, or the size of the bowl of a spoon. If you usually eat with a big spoon, try a smaller one and see if it changes the experience.

» Experiment with different music as you eat. Restaurants put a lot of thought into their playlists because it truly can heighten enjoyment.

» Plant something edible—even one small parsley seed in a little plastic container on your windowsill. This one might germinate, it might not—it's the process that matters, and seeing how hard it can be to grow food can increase your appreciation of it. As with everything in life, there is no failure here, only learning. And maybe you'll enjoy it so much it will turn into a hobby.

Blueberry (or Almost Any Berry) Crisp

Ideally you'll find all your food pleasurable, but sometimes you want something sweet and warm and doughy. This recipe gives sweetness and still provides some beneficial nutrients to support your mental health. If possible, get wild blueberries. They are extremely high in polyphenols, which support mental health (all blueberries have at least some of the flavonoid anthocyanin). Studies of anthocyanin, the pigment found in blueberries, show that it improves mood. There is evidence that blueberries can reduce inflammation and help with serotonin production. The gooey blueberries' sweetness is concentrated by baking, and it reminds me of the fruit-on-the-bottom sugary yogurt that I sometimes had in my youth—but better. Blueberry crisp will emotionally support you as you rise to the challenges of your life. The aroma of cinnamon is calming, and it's weirdly satisfying to put your fingers right in the topping to pinch it together. And it's versatile—you can use any berry on the bottom (anthocyanin is also found in blackberries and raspberries, so feel free to mix it up) and add nuts or spices to the topping, which is basically a big oatmeal cookie. This crisp works even for out-of-season fruit that is a little sour because cooking fruit caramelizes and intensifies its natural sugars. The topping is 100 percent whole grain and honey sweetened. I once made 300 samples of this on a brutally hot day at the White House Farmers' Market at a time when people at the White House needed a lot of calming. The samples were gone in 30 minutes.

SERVES 8

continued

⅔ cup whole wheat flour

1½ cups rolled oats

1 teaspoon kosher salt, divided

1 teaspoon cinnamon

½ cup olive oil

½ cup good honey

½ teaspoon vanilla

6 cups blueberries (or toss in any leftover berries rolling around in your refrigerator for a mixed fruit crisp)

2 teaspoons lemon juice

1 tablespoon chopped fresh mint

Heat oven to 350°F. Place the flour, oats, half the salt, and the cinnamon in a bowl and toss to combine. In a separate bowl, mix the oil, honey, and vanilla with a fork or a whisk until loosely mixed (it will probably not combine completely). Then pour the wet ingredients into the bowl with the dry ingredients and mix with your fingers to combine. In a 10-by-7-inch pan, place the blueberries and mix with the lemon juice and mint to combine. Top the blueberries with crumble mixture and sprinkle the remaining salt on top. Place the dish on a baking sheet (it may bubble over) and bake for about 50 minutes, until the blueberries have released their juices and the top of the oatmeal mixture browns. Let the crisp sit (if you can resist) for about half an hour (or more) at room temperature to let the blueberries set—otherwise it will be really liquidy, which is also delicious, just a different experience.

Five Ways to Practice the "How" of Mindful Eating in Real Life

It would be great if we could all pause, close our eyes, savor, and engage with all the other mindful things that people suggest (I have a feeling it's easier for them than it is for me). I once went on a retreat where mindful eating meals were offered—no talking or other distractions, just you and a meal. For every meal. Every day. For days. I actually wound up dreading mealtime because it became so tedious. If eating this way works for you, do it!

For the rest of us, here are some practical ideas for integrating mindful eating into our everyday lives:

1. **Don't eat in a car or while moving.** The average American eats one of every five meals in the car, and there is evidence that those meals don't register as pleasurable as meals eaten elsewhere. When your body is in motion, your brain is partially focused on the movement. Sit down, or at the very least stand still. Give your brain the best chance to actually enjoy the food you're ingesting, no matter what it is.

2. **Layer smells.** If you're eating food with some lime in it, try grating lime zest on top of your dish—there will be a lot of lime scent and a little extra taste too. If you're baking cookies, save a few bits of dough to pop in the oven when you serve the cookies—the smell will heighten the flavor. I sometimes put a small drop of good olive oil on a lamp lightbulb a few minutes before a meal—the heat from the bulb heightens the scent and tells my brain it's time for something good.

3. **Choose the communal table.** At some fast-food restaurants there are long tables for eight or more people—a space-saving way to offer more seating in a smaller space. Communal tables are often used for overflow seating when diners can't find a smaller table. Even if you're the only one in the restaurant, try sitting at the communal table, even if you're trying to work. Just being around others, even if you're not talking, can be beneficial.

4. **Put on some sounds you associate with what you're eating.** Try listening to the sound of waves crashing when eating seafood or a song that was popular when you were a teenager when having a childhood comfort food. Make eating playlists. If it works for highly rated restaurants, it may work for you at home.

5. **Give thanks.** Even a split second of recognition that you're grateful for sustenance of any kind can shift your mind to taste food differently. Remember, flavor is created in the brain and anything you do can heighten your pleasure.

Afterword

"Between stimulus and response there is a space.
In that space is our power to choose our response.
In our response lies our growth and freedom."
—VIKTOR FRANKL

EATING TO SUPPORT emotional well-being has changed my life. Making peace with my body is a top priority for me, to focus on its abilities rather than its drawbacks (things I see as drawbacks anyway—my appreciation for my own quirks has evolved alongside my eating).

I set my sights on eating to feel emotionally better, which for me has at least two meanings. First, that something formerly dampening my mood has lifted, that my emotions feel better than they did before. Second, that I have less difficulty with experiencing and processing emotions—I literally feel my emotions better, with improved and skillful flexibility.

When anxiety and fear come, I know what to look for in my mind and body. I recognize the thoughts that pop up in my mind and the physical effects they have. And I'm usually able to feel a difficult emotion and allow space between that feeling and my action. That action could be something I say or do in the world, or it could just be the default thoughts that come into my own head to interpret events. Those thoughts are just as important as immediate action; those thoughts will inform my future actions.

Paying attention to emotional eating has made me protective of my mental health in general, too, as I try to guard the virtuous cycle I've strived for. Making small efforts like the ones listed in Chapter 6 have reinforced my overall commitment to safeguarding myself. A lot has contributed to that—getting out of a bad relationship, having a great therapist, liking my job, general pandemic life reassessment.

So much of what I learned by poring over journal articles, visiting labs, and talking to researchers around the globe has worked in my own life. You've heard the saying, "It's not the destination but the journey that matters"? I think with emotional well-being the journey *is* the destination. We try every day to experience emotional well-being while we simultaneously try to develop greater abilities for our future selves. We build the airplane while it's flying in midair. It's, maybe not coincidentally, the same thing with cooking.

I think often about the feast paradox—that people who eat together eat food (which we often associate with poor health) but have better health. Usually I'll recall this paradox when I'm in the office and have an impulse to just sit at my desk and work through lunch. It's sometimes easier to burrow into work than to risk bringing my messiness to a table with people. But even if it's for just five or ten minutes, I go from the newsroom to the lunchroom. And we eat together. The experience is not always transforming, but it's always worthwhile because it's part of a pattern. Relationships, even the five-minute ones in the lunchroom, are all part of emotional well-being.

On most days, I eat mostly whole foods and heaps of vegetables, way more than I used to. Ultra-processed food is no longer part of my mindless eating pattern—my default foods tend to be on the nuts and yogurt side of the spectrum. I count fiber and fermented foods, not calories. I experimented with different cutlery for my home until I found utensils that are pleasing to look at, hold, and put in my mouth—I particularly love the feeling of the bowl of the spoon.

I grow Thai basil year-round, either indoors or outside. I use it in almost everything that calls for regular basil; the complexity of Thai basil just adds another dimension (don't tell my Italian ancestors). It can be expensive and hard to find, so the little bit of time I put into growing it is a net win. I have a potted dwarf citrus tree indoors that thrives even in winter—it's not practically useful, but I love seeing citrus growing when it snows outside. It reminds me that spring is always coming.

I live my priority of protecting my mental health by cooking and eating with a new "why" now. Why cook? Why eat whole foods? I eat and cook to help me live a better emotional life, to feel better, including immense and intense pleasure along the way. I spent so much time fighting with my body and the biological realities of emotional eating. Eating for emotional well-being is my now powerful and gentle "why."

Acknowledgments

I'VE READ THAT some writers identify their dream editors by searching the acknowledgment sections of beloved books. If you're here for that reason, I can tell you that Ann Triestman is the best—an empathic and realistic editor who has become a friend and fellow eating-for-emotional-well-being traveler. I'm so fortunate that she, and the Countryman team, are my partners in bringing the science to readers hungry (*haha*) for ways to eat for both health and pleasure. Alongside Ann, Devorah Backman is a true believer in this work and is tireless in her efforts to put it out into the world. Thanks to my team of amazing women who champion the power of food to improve the human experience, including literary agent Bridget Matzie, publicist Deb Shapiro, and Anna Jinks at CAA. I'm so grateful.

This book's existence depended on the dozens of scientists, researchers, physicians, and chefs who gave me their time for interviews. It's only through this kind of generous collaboration that we can all touch different parts of the animal and finally figure out it's an elephant.

My son, Truman, just by being himself, is a constant wonder and inspiration. Of all the lucky things in my life, the luckiest may be that he is surrounded by supportive and smart people at Episcopal High School in Virginia—especially Kadeem Rodgers, who knows how to prioritize being the best human and player you can be (in that order) and helps me to understand the transformative value of sports. Also, because he encourages eating vegetables. Back in the 1980s, my elementary school teachers at

Center School in New Canaan, Connecticut, had us turn our writing into books, with cardboard covers decorated with old wallpaper samples. What we tell young people about their value, and what we funnel into children's imaginations, matters—for the child and the world.

Thank you to Allen, Jen, and Heather Koop, who continue to count me as family long after Chick and Betty were gone. And they're not really gone—when *Eat & Flourish* was translated into Japanese, I put a copy on my bookshelf right next to the biography of my mentor C. Everett Koop, in Japanese. I remember seeing that copy when I was in my early twenties and thinking, *Wow, how great would it be to write something that is translated into other languages?* I am still pinching myself.

Eat & Flourish is dedicated to my sisters, so here is my double-thanks to them and their wonderful families. When children grow up with significant trauma, they can band together to validate the truth or, often, they break apart. My sisters and I continue to stand with each other, especially in the midst of complications from my father's recent death. I'm grateful I was able to read aloud to my father, minutes before he died, the parts of this book about his grandmother's cooking. Life is complicated and beautiful.

Love and infinite thanks to the Russos, for believing in my work and for sharing two places with me that I love so much I consider them homes: New York and Los Angeles. I am indebted to them, the Orient Village community, and people on the North Fork of Long Island (if you know, you know) for peaceful writing spaces. Writing about oysters while watching them being harvested in your backyard is a ridiculous privilege.

Truman, I love you no matter what. Thank you for helping me understand unconditional love—I'm not sure I believed in it before you were born. The world is a better place with you in it. Let your honesty shine and go live your one wild and precious life. You've got this. Trust me.

Notes

Introduction

Dunbar, RIM. Breaking bread: The functions of social eating. *Adapt Human Behav Physiol.* 2017; 3: 198–211. DOI: 10.1007/s40750-017-0061-4.

Freeman MP, Hibbeln JR, Wisner KL, et al. Omega-3 fatty acids: Evidence basis for treatment and future research in psychiatry. *J Clin Psychiatry.* 2006 Dec; 67(12): 1954–1967. DOI: 10.4088/jcp.v67n1217. Erratum in: *J Clin Psychiatry.* 2007 Feb; 68(2): 338. PMID: 17194275.

Kiecolt-Glaser JK, Belury MA, Andridge R, et al. Omega-3 supplementation lowers inflammation and anxiety in medical students: a randomized controlled trial. *Brain Behav Immun.* 2011 Nov.; 25(8): 1725–1734. DOI: 10.1016/j.bbi.2011.07.229. Epub 2011 Jul 19. PMID: 21784145; PMCID: PMC3191260.

Ljungberg T, Bondza E, Lethin C. Evidence of the importance of dietary habits regarding depressive symptoms and depression. *Int J Environ Res Public Health.* 2020; 17(5): 1616. Published 2020 Mar 2. DOI: 10.3390/ijerph17051616.

Needham DB, M, Adame MD, et al. A gut-derived metabolite alters brain activity and anxiety behaviour in mice. *Nature.* 2022. DOI: 10.1038/s41586-022-04396-8.

Radavelli-Bagatini S, Blekkenhorst LC, Sim M, et al. Fruit and vegetable intake is inversely associated with perceived stress across the adult lifespan. *Clin Nutr.* 2021 May; 40(5): 2860–2867. DOI: 10.1016/j.clnu.2021.03.043. Epub 2021 Apr 15. PMID: 33940399.

CHAPTER 1: Emotional Eating

Adan RAH, van der Beek EM, Buitelaar JK, et al. Nutritional psychiatry: Towards improving mental health by what you eat. *Eur Neuropsychopharmacol.* 2019 Dec; 29(12): 1321–32. DOI: 10.1016/j.euroneuro.2019.10.011. Epub 2019 Nov 14. PMID: 31735529.

Allen A, Hutch W, Borre Y, et al. *Bifidobacterium longum* 1714 as a translational psychobiotic:

Modulation of stress, electrophysiology and neurocognition in healthy volunteers. *Transl Psychiatry.* 2016; 6: e939. DOI: 10.1038/tp.2016.191.

Beilharz JE, Maniam J, Morris MJ. Short exposure to a diet rich in both fat and sugar or sugar alone impairs place, but not object recognition memory in rats. *Brain Behav Immun.* 2014 Mar; 37: 134–41. DOI: 10.1016/j.bbi.2013.11.016.

Betley J, Xu S, Cao Z, et al. Neurons for hunger and thirst transmit a negative-valence teaching signal. *Nature.* 2015; 521: 180–85. DOI: 10.1038/nature14416.

Chen H, Dunk MM, Wang B, et al. Associations of the Mediterranean-DASH Intervention for Neurodegenerative Delay diet with brain structural markers and their changes. *Alzheimers Dement.* 2023; 1–11. DOI: 10.1002/alz.13521.

Cho S, Kim S. Does a healthy lifestyle matter? A daily diary study of unhealthy eating at home and behavioral outcomes at work. *J Appl Psychol.* 2022 Jan; 107(1): 23–39. DOI: 10.1037/apl0000890. Epub 2021 Mar 25. PMID: 33764080.

Desai MS, Seekatz AM, Koropatkin NM, et al. A dietary fiber-deprived gut microbiota degrades the colonic mucus barrier and enhances pathogen susceptibility. *Cell.* 2016 Nov 17; 167(5): 1339–53. DOI: 10.1016/j.cell.2016.10.043.

Edwards LM, Murray AJ, Holloway CJ, et al. Short-term consumption of a high-fat diet impairs whole-body efficiency and cognitive function in sedentary men. *FASEB J.* 2011 Mar; 25(3): 1088–96. DOI: 10.1096/fj.10-171983. Epub 2010 Nov 24. PMID: 21106937.

Estruch R, Ros E, Salas-Salvadó J, et al. Primary prevention of cardiovascular disease with a Mediterranean diet supplemented with extra-virgin olive oil or nuts. *N Engl J Med.* 2018; 378: e34. DOI: 10.1056/NEJMoa1800389.

Firth J, Marx W, Dash S, et al. The effects of dietary improvement on symptoms of depression and anxiety: A meta-analysis of randomized controlled trials. *Psychosom Med.* 2019; 81(3): 265–80. DOI: 10.1097/PSY.0000000000000673. Published correction appears in *Psychosom Med.* 2020 Jun; 82(5): 536; published correction appears in *Psychosom Med.* 2021 Feb–Mar 01; 83(2): 196.

Francis HM, Stevenson RJ, Chambers JR, et al. A brief diet intervention can reduce symptoms of depression in young adults: A randomised controlled trial. *PLoS One.* 2019; 14(10): e0222768. DOI: 10.1371/journal.pone.0222768.

Gómez-Pinilla F. Brain foods: The effects of nutrients on brain function. *Nat Rev Neurosci.* 2008 Jul; 9(7): 568–78. DOI: 10.1038/nrn2421.

Hendy HM. Which comes first in food–mood relationships, foods or moods? *Appetite.* 2012; 58(2): 771–75. DOI: 10.1016/j.appet.2011.11.014.

Jack RE, Garrod OGB, Schyns PG. Dynamic facial expression of emotion transmit an evolving hierarchy of signals over time. *Curr Biol.* 2014; 24(2): 187–92. DOI: 10.1016/j.cub.2013.11.064.

Jacka FN, Cherbuin N, Anstey KJ, et al. Western diet is associated with a smaller hippocampus: A longitudinal investigation. *BMC Med.* 2015; 13: 215. DOI: 10.1186/s12916-015-0461-x.

Jacka FN, Mykletun A, Berk M, et al. The association between habitual diet quality and the common mental disorders in community-dwelling adults: The Hordaland Health study. *Psychosom Med.* 2011 Jul; 73(6): 483–90. DOI: 10.1097/PSY.0b013e318222831a.

Jacka FN, O'Neil A, Opie R, et al. A randomised controlled trial of dietary improvement for adults with major depression (the "SMILES" trial). *BMC Med.* 2017 Jan;15–23. DOI: 10.1186/s12916-017-0791-y.

Jacka FN, Pasco JA, Mykletun A, et al. Association of Western and traditional diets with depression and anxiety in women. *Am J Psych.* 2010 Mar; 167(3): 305–11. DOI: 10.1176/appi.ajp.2009.09060881.

Ke S, Wang XW, Ratanatharathorn A, et al. Association of probable post-traumatic stress disorder with dietary pattern and gut microbiome in a cohort of women. *Nature Mental Health.* 2023; 1: 900–13. DOI: 10.1038/s44220-023-00145-6.

Khanna P, Chattu VK, Aeri BT. Nutritional aspects of depression in adolescents: A systematic review. *Int J Prev Med.* 2019 Apr 3;10: 42. DOI: 10.4103/ijpvm.IJPVM-400-18.

Kohn R, Saxena S, Levav I, et al. The treatment gap in mental health care. *Bull World Health Organ.* 2004 Nov; 82(11): 858–66. Epub 2004 Dec 14. PMID: 15640922; PMCID: PMC2623050.

Kringelbach ML. The pleasure of food: Underlying brain mechanisms of eating and other pleasures. *Flavour.* 2015; 4(20). DOI: 10.1186/s13411-014-0029-2.

Labroo AA, Mukhopadhyay A. Lay theories of emotion transience and the search for happiness: A fresh perspective on affect regulation. *J Consum Res.* 2009 Aug; 36(2): 242–54. DOI: 10.1086/597159.

LaChance L, Aucoin M, Cooley K. Design and pilot evaluation of an evidence-based worksheet and clinician guide to facilitate nutrition counselling for patients with severe mental illness. *BMC Psychiatry.* 2021; 21: 556. DOI: 10.1186/s12888-021-03575-7.

Lassale C, Batty GD, Baghdadli A, et al. Healthy dietary indices and risk of depressive outcomes: A systematic review and meta-analysis of observational studies. *Mol Psychiatry.* 2019; 24; 965–86. DOI: 10.1038/s41380-018-0237-8.

Li Y, Lv MR, Wei YJ, et al. Dietary patterns and depression risk: A meta-analysis. *Psychiat Res.* 2017; 253: 373–82. DOI: 10.1016/j.psychres.2017.04.020.

Logan AC, Jacka FN. Nutritional psychiatry research: An emerging discipline and its intersection with global urbanization, environmental challenges, and the evolutionary mismatch. *J Physiol Anthropol.* 2014; 33(1): 22. DOI: 10.1186/1880-6805-33-22.

Navarro AM, Abasheva D, Martínez-González MÁ, et al. Coffee consumption and the risk of depression in a middle-aged cohort: The SUN Project. *Nutrients.* 2018 Sep 19; 10(9): 1333. DOI: 10.3390/nu10091333. PMID: 30235886; PMCID: PMC6163886.

Nonaka S, Arai C, Takayama M, et al. Efficient increase of γ-aminobutyric acid (GABA) content in tomato fruits by targeted mutagenesis. *Sci Rep.* 2017; 7(7057). DOI: 10.1038/s41598-017-06400-y.

O'Mahony SM, Clarke G, Borre YE, et al. Serotonin, tryptophan metabolism and the brain-gut-microbiome axis. *Behav Brain Res.* 2015 Jan 15; 277: 32–48. DOI: 10.1016/j.bbr.2014.07.027. Epub 2014 Jul 29. PMID: 25078296.

Opie RS, Ball K, Abbott G, et al. Adherence to the Australian dietary guidelines and development of depressive symptoms at 5 years follow-up amongst women in the READI cohort study. *Nutr J.* 2020; 19(30). DOI: 10.1186/s12937-020-00540-0.

Opie RS, Itsiopoulos C, Parletta N, et al. Dietary recommendations for the pre-vention of depression. *Nutr Neurosci.* 2017 Apr; 20(3): 161–71. DOI: 10.1179/1476830515Y.0000000043. Epub 2016 Mar 2. PMID: 26317148.

Owen L, Corfe B. The role of diet and nutrition on mental health and wellbeing. *Proc Nutr Soc.* 2017 Nov; 76(4): 425–26. DOI: 10.1017/S0029665117001057. Epub 2017 Jul 14. PMID: 28707609.

Parletta N, Zarnowiecki D, Cho J, et al. A Mediterranean-style intervention supplemented with fish oil improves diet quality and mental health in people with depression: A ran-domized controlled trial (HELFIMED). *Nutr Neurosci.* 2019; 22(7): 474–87. DOI: 10.1080/1028415X.2017.1411320.

Ravindran AV, Balneaves LG, Faulkner G, et al. Canadian Network for Mood and Anxiety Treatments (CANMAT) 2016 Clinical Guidelines for the Management of Adults with Major Depressive Disorder: Section 5. Complementary and Alternative Medicine Treat-ments. *Can J Psychiatry.* 2016; 61(9): 576–87. DOI: 10.1177/0706743716660290.

Sánchez-Villegas A, Delgado-Rodríguez M, Alonso A, et al. Association of the Mediterra-nean dietary pattern with the incidence of depression: The Seguimiento Universidad de Navarra/University of Navarra follow-up (SUN) cohort. *Arch Gen Psychiatry.* 2009 Oct; 66(10): 1090–8. DOI: 10.1001/archgenpsychiatry.2009.129. PMID: 19805699.

Sánchez-Villegas A, Martinéz-González MA, Estruch R, et al. Mediterranean dietary pattern and depression: The PREDIMED randomized trial. *BMC Med.* 2013 Sep; 11: 208. DOI: 10.1186/1741-7015-11-208.

Sánchez-Villegas A, Verberne L, Da Irala J, et al. Dietary fat intake and the risk of depression: The SUN study. *PLoS One.* 2011 Jan; 6(1) :e16268. DOI: 10.1371/journal.pone.0016268.

Sarris J, Logan AC, Akbaraly T, et al. International Society for Nutritional Psychiatry Research consensus position statement: Nutritional medicine in modern psychiatry. *World Psychiatry.* 2015 Oct; 14(3): 370–1. DOI: 10.1002/wps.20223.

Sarris J, Logan AC, Akbaraly T, et al. Nutritional medicine as mainstream in psychiatry. *Lan-cet Psychiatry.* 2015 Mar; 2(3): 271–74. DOI: 10.1016/S2215-0366(14)00051-0.

Sathyanarayana Rao TS, Asha MR, Ramesh BN, et al. Understanding nutrition, depression, and mental illness. *Indian J Psychiatry.* 2008 Jun; 50(2): 77–82. DOI: 10.4103/0019-5545.42391.

Savignac HM, Kiely B, Dinan TG, et al. *Bifidobacteria* exert strain-specific effects on stress-related behavior and physiology in BALB/c mice. *Neurogastroenterol Motil.* 2014 Nov; 26(11): 1615–27. DOI: 10.1111/nmo.12427. Epub 2014 Sep 24. PMID: 25251188.

Stahl ST, Albert SM, Dew MA, et al Coaching in healthy dietary practices in at-risk older adults: A case of indicated depression prevention. *Am J Psychiatry.* 2014; 171(5): 499–505. DOI: 10.1176/appi.ajp.2013.13101373.

Tian P, Bastiaanssen TFS, Song L, et al. Unraveling the microbial mechanisms underlying the psychobiotic potential of a *Bifidobacterium breve* strain. *Mol Nutr Food Res.* 2021 Apr; 65(8): e2000704. DOI: 10.1002/mnfr.202000704. Epub 2021 Mar 9. PMID: 33594816.

Waters SF, Karnilowicz HR, West TV, et al. Keep it to yourself? Parent emotion suppression influences physiological linkage and interaction behavior. *J Fam Psychol*. 2020 Oct; 34(7): 784–93. DOI: 10.1037/fam0000664. Epub 2020 Apr 23. PMID: 32324017.

Wee RWS, Mishchanchuk K, AlSubaie R, et al. Internal-state-dependent control of feeding behavior via hippocampal ghrelin signaling. *Neuron*. 2023; 112(2): 228–305. DOI: 10.1016/j.neuron.2023.10.016.

Wickham SR, Amarasekara NA, Bartonicek A, et al. The big three health behaviors and mental health and well-being among young adults: A cross-sectional investigation of sleep, exercise, and diet. *Front Psychol*. 2020 Dec 10; 11: 579205. DOI: 10.3389/fpsyg.2020.579205. PMID: 33362643; PMCID: PMC7758199.

Yang C, Fujita Y, Ren Q, et al. *Bifidobacterium* in the gut microbiota confer resilience to chronic social defeat stress in mice. *Sci Rep*. 2017; 7: 45942. DOI: 10.1038/srep45942.

Zhang X, Wang H, Kilpatrick LA, et al. Discrimination exposure impacts unhealthy processing of food cues: crosstalk between the brain and gut. *Nature Mental Health*. 2023; 1: 841–52. DOI: 10.1038/s44220-023-00134-9.

Zhao J, Zhao N. The links between food components, dietary habits, and gut microbiota composition. *Foods*. 2023; 12(20): 3780. DOI: 10.3390/foods12203780.

Zou J, Chassaing B, Singh V, et al. Fiber-mediated nourishment of gut microbiota protects against diet-induced obesity by restoring IL-22 mediated colonic health. *Cell Host Microbe*. 2018; 23: 41–53. DOI: 10.1016/j.chom.2017.11.003.

CHAPTER 2: Pleasure

Castro B, Berridge K. Opioid and orexin hedonic hotspots in rat orbitofrontal cortex and insula. *Proc Natl Acad Sci USA*. 2017 Oct; 114(43): 201705753. DOI: 10.1073/pnas.1705753114.

Chalmin-Pui L, Griffiths A, Roe J, et al. Why garden? Attitudes and the perceived health benefits of home gardening. *Cities*. 2021; 112: 103118. DOI: 10.1016/j.cities.2021.103118.

Deblais A, Hollander ED, Boucon C, et al. Predicting thickness perception of liquid food products from their non-Newtonian rheology. *Nat Commun*. 2021 Nov 3; 12(1): 6328. DOI: 10.1038/s41467-021-26687-w.

Dess NK, Edelheit D. The bitter with the sweet: The taste/stress/temperament nexus. *Biol Psychol*. 1998 June; 48(2): 103–19. DOI: 10.1016/s0301-0511(98)00014-3. PMID: 9700013.

Dijker AJ. Moderate eating with pleasure and without effort: Toward understanding the underlying psychological mechanisms. *Health Psychol Open*. 2019; 6(2): 2055102919889883. Published 2019 Nov 21. DOI: 10.1177/2055102919889883.

Drewnowski A, Almiron-Roig E. "Human Perceptions and Preferences for Fat-Rich Foods." In Montmayeur JP, le Coutre J, editors. *Fat Detection: Taste, Texture, and Post Ingestive Effects*, (2010). Boca Raton, FL: CRC Press/Taylor & Francis. Chapter 11. Available from: https://www.ncbi.nlm.nih.gov/books/NBK53528/.

Dunbar, RIM. Breaking bread: The functions of social eating. *Adapt Human Behav Physiol*. 2017; 3: 198–211. DOI: 10.1007/s40750-017-0061-4.

Fanzo J, Rudie C, Sigman I, et al. Sustainable food systems and nutrition in the 21st century: A report from the 22nd annual Harvard Nutrition Obesity Symposium. *Am J Clin Nutr.* 2022 Jan 11; 115(1): 18–33. DOI: 10.1093/ajcn/nqab315. PMID: 34523669; PMCID: PMC8755053.

Farmer N, Touchton-Leonard K, Ross A. Psychosocial benefits of cooking interventions: A systematic review. *Health Educ Behav.* 2018 Apr; 45(2): 167–80. DOI: 10.1177/1090198117736352. Epub 2017 Nov 9. PMID: 29121776; PMCID: PMC5862744.

Global Child Nutrition Foundation (GCNF). 2022. *School Meal Programs Around the World: Results from the 2021 Global Survey of School Meal Programs.*

Hamburg ME, Finkenauer C, Schuengel C. Food for love: The role of food offering in empathic emotion regulation. *Front Psychol.* 2014 Jan 31; 5: 32. DOI: 10.3389/fpsyg.2014.00032.

Hayashi LC, Benasi G, St-Onge MP, et al. Intuitive and mindful eating to improve physiological health parameters: A short narrative review of intervention studies. *J Complement Integr Med.* 2021 Dec 16. DOI: 10.1515/jcim-2021-0294.

Heath TP, Melichar JK, Nutt DJ, et al. Human taste thresholds are modulated by serotonin and noradrenaline. *J Neurosci.* 2006 Dec 6; 26(49): 12664–71. DOI: 10.1523/JNEUROSCI.3459-06.2006. PMID: 17151269; PMCID: PMC6674841.

Howell RT, Chenot D, Hill G, et al. Momentary happiness: The role of psychological need satisfaction." *J Happiness Stud.* 2011; 12: 1–15. DOI: 10.1007/s10902-009-9166-1.

Jeans MR, Landry MJ, Vandyousefi S, et al. Effects of a school-based gardening, cooking, and nutrition cluster randomized controlled trial on unprocessed and ultraprocessed food consumption. *J Nutr.* 2023; 153(7): 2073–84. DOI: 10.1016/j.tjnut.2023.04.013.

Leonard BE. The olfactory bulbectomized rat as a model of depression. *Pol J Pharmacol Pharm.* 1984; 36(5): 561–69.

Li S, Li R, Hu X, et al. Omega-3 supplementation improves depressive symptoms, cognitive function, and niacin skin flushing response in adolescent depression: A randomized controlled clinical trial. *J Affect Disord.* 2024; 345: 394–403. DOI: 10.1016/j.jad.2023.10.151.

Losecaat Vermeer AB, Muth A, Terenzi D, et al. Curiosity for information predicts wellbeing mediated by loneliness during COVID-19 pandemic. *Sci Rep.* 2022; 12: 7771. DOI: 10.1038/s41598-022-11924-z.

Luo Y, Chen X, Qi S, et al. Well-being and anticipation for future positive events: Evidences from an fMRI study. *Front Psychol.* 2018; 8: 2199. DOI: 10.3389/fpsyg.2017.02199.

Miller RK, Luckemeyer TJ, Kerth CR, et al. Descriptive beef flavor and texture attributes relationships with consumer acceptance of US light beef eaters. *Meat Sci.* 2023; 204: 109252. DOI: 10.1016/j.meatsci.2023.109252.

O'Mahoney SM, Clarke G, Borre YE, et al. Serotonin, tryptophan metabolism and the brain-gut-microbiome axis. *Behav Brain Res.* 2015 Jan; 277: 32–48. DOI: 10.1016/j.bbr.2014.07.027.

Platte P, Herbert C, Pauli P, et al. Oral perceptions of fat and taste stimuli are modulated by affect and mood induction. *PLoS One*. 2013 June 5; 8(6): e65006. DOI: 10.1371/journal .pone.0065006. PMID: 23755167; PMCID: PMC3673997.

Porter J, Craven B, Khan RM, et al. Mechanisms of scent-tracking in humans. *Nat Neurosci*. 2007 Jan; 10(1): 27–9. DOI: 10.1038/nn1819. Epub 2006 Dec 17. Erratum in *Nat Neurosci*. 2007 Feb; 10(2): 263. Judkewicz, Benjamin [corrected to Judkewitz, Benjamin]. PMID: 17173046.

Ratcliffe E, Baxter WL, Martin N. Consumption rituals relating to food and drink: A review and research agenda. *Appetite*. 2019 Mar 1; 134: 86–93. DOI: 10.1016/j.appet.2018.12.021. Epub 2018 Dec 17. PMID: 30572007.

Shanahan LK, Bhutani S, Kahnt T. Olfactory perceptual decision-making is biased by motivational state. *PLoS Biol*. 2021 Aug 26; 19(8): e3001374. DOI: 10.1371/journal .pbio.3001374. PMID: 34437533; PMCID: PMC8389475.

Smith-Carrier TA, Béres L, Johnson K, et al. Digging into the experiences of therapeutic gardening for people with dementia: An interpretative phenomenological analysis. *Dementia (London)*. 2021 Jan; 20(1): 130–47. DOI: 10.1177/1471301219869121. Epub 2019 Aug 19. PMID: 31426675.

Spence, C. Comfort food: A review. *Int J Gastron Food Sci*. 2017; 9: 105–9.

Spence, C. Unraveling the mystery of the rounder, sweeter chocolate bar. *Flavour*. 2013; 2: 28. DOI: 10.1186/2044-7248-2-28.

Spence C, Mancini M, Huisman G. Digital commensality: Eating and drinking in the company of technology. *Front Psychol*. 2019 Oct 9; 10: 2252. DOI: 10.3389/fpsyg.2019 .02252.

Spence C, Youssef J. Olfactory dining: Designing for the dominant sense. *Flavour*. 2015; 4: 32. DOI: 10.1186/s13411-015-0042-0.

Stice E, Burger KS, Yokum S. Reward region responsivity predicts future weight gain and moderating effects of the *TaqIA* allele. *J Neurosci*. 2015 Jul 15; 35(28): 10316–24. DOI: 10.1523/JNEUROSCI.3607-14.2015. PMID: 26180206; PMCID: PMC4502268.

Stice E, Yokum S. Effects of gymnemic acids lozenge on reward region response to receipt and anticipated receipt of high-sugar food. *Physiol Behav*. 2018 Oct 1; 194: 568–76. DOI: 10.1016/j.physbeh.2018.07.012. Epub 2018 Jul 20. PMID: 30031752.

Stice E, Yokum S, Burger K, et al. A pilot randomized trial of a cognitive reappraisal obesity prevention program. *Physiol Behav*. 2015 Jan; 138: 124–32. DOI: 10.1016/j.physbeh.2014.10.022. Epub 2014 Oct 30. PMID: 25447334; PMCID: PMC4258533.

Stice E, Yokum S, Veling H, et al. Pilot test of a novel food response and attention training treatment for obesity: Brain imaging data suggest actions shape valuation. *Behav Res Ther*. 2017 Jul; 94: 60–70. DOI: 10.1016/j.brat.2017.04.007. Epub 2017 Apr 19. PMID: 28505470; PMCID: PMC5656010.

Tian AD, Schroeder J, Häubl G, et al. Enacting rituals to improve self-control. *J Pers Soc Psychol*. 2018; 114(6): 851–76. DOI: 10.1037/pspa0000113.

Vignolles A, Pichon PE. A taste of nostalgia: Links between nostalgia and food consumption. *Qualitative Market Research: An International Journal.* 2014; 17: 10. DOI: 1108/ QMR-06-2012-0027.

Vohs KD, Wang Y, Gino F, et al. Rituals enhance consumption. *Psychol Sci.* 2013; 24(9): 1714–21. DOI: 10.1177/0956797613478949.

Wagner HS, Ahlstrom B, Redden JP, et al. The myth of comfort food. *Health Psychol.* 2014 Dec; 33(12): 1552–57. DOI: 10.1037/hea0000068. Epub 2014 Aug 18. PMID: 25133833.

Zahedi H, Djalalinia S, Sadeghi O, et al. Breakfast consumption and mental health: A systematic review and meta-analysis of observational studies. *Nutr Neurosci.* 2020: 1250–64. DOI: 10.1080/1028415X.2020.1853411.

CHAPTER 3: The Gut Microbiome

Bahar RJ, Collins BS, Steinmetz B, et al. Double-blind placebo-controlled trial of amitriptyline for the treatment of irritable bowel syndrome in adolescents. *J Pediatr.* 2008 May; 152(5): 685–89. DOI: 10.1016/j.jpeds.2007.10.012. Epub 2008 Feb 20. PMID: 18410774.

Bastiaanssen TFS, Cryan JF. Dairy alters the microbiome, are we but skimming the surface? *EBioMedicine.* 2021 Jun; 68: 103417. DOI: 10.1016/j.ebiom.2021.103417. Epub 2021 Jun 3. PMID: 34091415; PMCID: PMC8185236.

Bercik P, Denou E, Collins J, et al. The intestinal microbiota affect central levels of brain-derived neurotropic factor and behavior in mice. *Gastroenterology.* 2011 Aug; 141(2): 599–609, 609.e1–3. DOI: 10.1053/j.gastro.2011.04.052. Epub 2011 Apr 30. PMID: 21683077.

Berding K, Cryan JF. Microbiota-targeted interventions for mental health. *Curr Opin Psychiatry.* 2022; 35(1): 3–9. DOI:10.1097/YCO.0000000000000758.

Boehme M, Guzzetta KE, Bastiaanssen TFS, et al. Microbiota from young mice counteracts selective age-associated behavioral deficits. *Nat Aging.* 2021; 1: 666–76. DOI: 10.1038/ s43587-021-00093-9.

Boscaini S, Leigh SJ, Lavelle A, et al. Microbiota and body weight control: Weight watchers within? *Mol Metab.* 2022 Mar; 57: 101427. DOI: 10.1016/j.molmet.2021.101427. Epub 2021 Dec 29. PMID: 34973469; PMCID: PMC8829807.

Bull MJ, Plummer NT. Part 1: The human gut microbiome in health and disease. *Integr Med (Encinitas).* 2014; 13(6): 17–22.

Chevalier G, Siopi E, Guenin-Macé L, et al. Effect of gut microbiota on depressive-like behaviors in mice is mediated by the endocannabinoid system. *Nat Commun.* 2020; 11: 6363. DOI: 10.1038/s41467-020-19931-2.

David LA, Maurice CF, Carmody RN, et al. Diet rapidly and reproducibly alters the human gut microbiome. *Nature.* 2014 Jan 23; 505(7484): 559–63. DOI: 10.1038/nature12820. Epub 2013 Dec 11. PMID: 24336217; PMCID: PMC3957428.

Davis CD. The gut microbiome and its role in obesity. *Nutr Today.* 2016; 51(4): 167–74. DOI: 10.1097/NT.0000000000000167.

Dickerson F, Adamos M, Katsafanas E, et al. Adjunctive probiotic microorganisms to prevent rehospitalization in patients with acute mania: A randomized controlled trial. *Bipolar*

Disord. 2018 Nov; 20(7): 614–21. DOI: 10.1111/bdi.12652. Epub 2018 Apr 25. PMID: 29693757.

Goodrich JK, Waters JL, Poole AC, et al. Human genetics shape the gut microbiome. *Cell.* 2014; 159(4): 789–99. DOI: 10.1016/j.cell.2014.09.053.

Graf D, Di Cagno R, Fåk F, et al. Contribution of diet to the composition of the human gut microbiota. *Microb Ecol Health Dis.* 2015 Feb 4; 26: 26164. DOI: 10.3402/mehd .v26.26164.

Klunemann M, Andrejev S, Blasch S, et al. Bioaccumulation of therapeutic drugs by human gut bacteria. *Nature.* 2021 Sep; 597: 533–38. DOI: 10.1038/s41586-021-03891-8.

Krajmalnik-Brown R, Ilhan ZE, Kang DW, et al. Effects of gut microbes on nutrient absorption and energy regulation. *Nutr Clin Pract.* 2012 Apr; 27(2): 201–14. DOI: 10.1177/088453361 1436116. Epub 2012 Feb 24. PMID: 22367888; PMCID: PMC3601187.

Leeming ER, Johnson AJ, Spector TD, et al. Effect of diet on the gut microbiota: Rethinking intervention duration. *Nutrients.* 2019 Nov 22; 11(12): 2862. DOI: 10.3390/nu11122862. PMID: 31766592; PMCID: PMC6950569.

Leitão-Gonçalves R, Carvalho-Santos Z, Francisco AP, et al. Commensal bacteria and essential amino acids control food choice behavior and reproduction. *PLoS Biol.* 2017 Apr 25; 15(4): e2000862. DOI: 10.1371/journal.pbio.2000862. PMID: 28441450; PMCID: PMC5404834.

Lewis CM Jr, Obregón-Tito A, Tito RY, et al. The Human Microbiome Project: Lessons from human genomics. *Trends Microbiol.* 2012 Jan; 20(1): 1–4. DOI: 10.1016/j .tim.2011.10.004. Epub 2011 Nov 21. PMID: 22112388; PMCID: PMC3709440.

Limbana T, Khan F, Eskander N. Gut microbiome and depression: How microbes affect the way we think. *Cureus.* 2020 Aug 23; 12(8): e9966. DOI: 10.7759/cureus.9966.

Liu RT, Walsh RFL, Sheehan AE. Prebiotics and probiotics for depression and anxiety: A systematic review and meta-analysis of controlled clinical trials. *Neurosci Biobehav Rev.* 2019 July; 102: 13–23. DOI: 10.1016/j.neubiorev.2019.03.023. Epub 2019 Apr 17. PMID: 31004628; PMCID: PMC6584030.

Martin CR, Osadchiy V, Kalani A, et al. The brain-gut-microbiome axis. *Cell Mol Gastroenterol Hepatol.* 2018 Apr 12; 6(2): 133–48. DOI: 10.1016/j.jcmgh.2018.04.003.

McDonald D, Hyde E, Debelius JW, et al. American gut: An open platform for citizen science microbiome research. *mSystems.* 2018 May 15; 3(3): e00031–18. DOI: 10.1128/mSystems .00031-18. PMID: 29795809; PMCID: PMC5954204.

Miller I. The gut-brain axis: Historical reflections. *Microb Ecol Health Dis.* 2018 Nov 8; 29(1): 1542921. DOI: 10.1080/16512235.2018.1542921.

Morais LH, Golubeva AV, Casey S, et al. Early-life oxytocin attenuates the social deficits induced by caesarean-section delivery in the mouse. *Neuropsychopharmacol.* 2021; 46: 1958–68. DOI: 10.1038/s41386-021-01040-3.

Navarro-Tapia E, Almeida-Toledano L, Sebastiani G, et al. Effects of microbiota imbalance in anxiety and eating disorders: Probiotics as novel therapeutic approaches. *Int J Mol Sci.* 2021 Feb 26; 22(5): 2351. DOI: 10.3390/ijms22052351. PMID: 33652962; PMCID: PMC7956573.

Ng QX, Peters C, Ho CYX, et al. A meta-analysis of the use of probiotics to alleviate depressive symptoms. *J Affect Disord*. 2018 Mar 1; 228: 13–19. DOI: 10.1016/j.jad.2017.11.063. Epub 2017 Nov 16. PMID: 29197739.

Richards P, Thornberry NA, Pinto S. The gut-brain axis: Identifying new therapeutic approaches for type 2 diabetes, obesity, and related disorders. *Mol Metab*. 2021; 46: 101175. DOI:10.1016/j.molmet.2021.101175.

Rinninella E, Raoul P, Cintoni M, et al. What is the healthy gut microbiota composition? A changing ecosystem across age, environment, diet, and diseases. *Microorganisms*. 2019 Jan 10; 7(1): 14. DOI: 10.3390/microorganisms7010014.

Rook GA, Lowry CA, Raison CL. Microbial "old friends," immunoregulation and stress resilience. *Evol Med Public Health*. 2013 Jan; 2013(1): 46–64. DOI: 10.1093/emph/eot004. Epub 2013 Apr 9. PMID: 24481186; PMCID: PMC3868387.

Sarkar A, Lehto SM, Harty S, et al. Psychobiotics and the manipulation of bacteria-gut-brain signals. *Trends Neurosci*. 2016; 39(11): 763–81. DOI: 10.1016/j.tins.2016.09.002.

Savignac HM, Kiely B, Dinan TG, et al. *Bifidobacteria* exert strain-specific effects on stress-related behavior and physiology in BALB/c mice. *Neurogastroenterol Motil*. 2014 Nov; 26(11): 1615-27. DOI: 10.1111/nmo.12427. Epub 2014 Sep 24. PMID: 25251188.

Spencer CN, McQuade JL, Gopalakrishnan V, et al. Dietary fiber and probiotics influence the gut microbiome and melanoma immunotherapy response. *Science*. 2021 Dec 24; 374(6575): 1632–40. DOI: 10.1126/science.aaz7015. Epub 2021 Dec 23. PMID: 34941392.

Thursby E, Juge N. Introduction to the human gut microbiota. *Biochem J*. 2017 May 16; 474(11): 1823–36. DOI: 10.1042/BCJ20160510.

Trevelline BK, Kohl KD. The gut microbiome influences host diet selection behavior. *Proc Natl Acad Sci USA*. 2022 Apr 19; 119(17): e2117537119. DOI: 10.1073/pnas.2117537119.

Turnbaugh PJ, Hamady M, Yatsunenko T, et al. A core gut microbiome in obese and lean twins. *Nature*. 2009 Jan 22; 457(7228): 480–84. DOI: 10.1038/nature07540. Epub 2008 Nov 30. PMID: 19043404; PMCID: PMC2677729.

Willyard C. How gut microbes could drive brain disorders. *Nature*. 2021 Feb; 590(7844): 22–25. DOI: 10.1038/d41586-021-00260-3. PMID: 33536656.

CHAPTER 4: **Inflammation**

American Psychological Association. *Stress in America 2020: Stress in the Time of Covid-19*. Stress in America Survey. 2020.

Basiri R, Seidu B, Cheskin LJ. Key nutrients for optimal blood glucose control and mental health in individuals with diabetes: A review of the evidence. *Nutrients*. 2023; 15(18): 3929. DOI: 10.3390/nu15183929.

Basiri R, Seidu B, Rudich M. Exploring the interrelationships between diabetes, nutrition, anxiety, and depression: Implications for treatment and prevention strategies. *Nutrients*. 2023; 15(19): 4226. DOI: 10.3390/nu15194226.

Baynham R, Weaver SRC, Rendeiro C, et al. Fat intake impairs the recovery of endothelial function following mental stress in young healthy adults. *Front. Nutr.* 2023; 10: 1275708. DOI: 10.3389/fnut.2023.1275708.

Breland JY, Donalson R, Dinh JV, et al. Trauma exposure and disordered eating: A qualitative study. *Women Health.* 2018 Feb; 58(2): 160–74. DOI: 10.1080/03630242.2017.1282398. Epub 2017 Feb 8. PMID: 28095133; PMCID: PMC6192417.

Chen GQ, Peng CL, Lian Y, et al. Association between dietary inflammatory index and mental health: A systematic review and dose—Response meta-analysis. *Front Nutr.* 5 May 2021; 8. DOI: 10.3389/fnut.2021.662357.

Cotter T, Kotov A, Wang S, et al. "Warning: ultra-processed": A call for warnings on foods that aren't really foods. *BMJ Glob Health.* 2021 Dec; 6(12): e007240. DOI: 10.1136/bmjgh-2021-007240. PMID: 34933866; PMCID: PMC8666852.

Davison KM, Hyland CE, West ML, et al. Post-traumatic stress disorder (PTSD) in mid-age and older adults differs by immigrant status and ethnicity, nutrition, and other determinants of health in the Canadian Longitudinal Study on Aging (CLSA). *Soc Psychiatry Psychiatr Epidemiol.* 2021; 56: 963–80. DOI: 10.1007/s00127-020-02003-7.

Fedorikhin A, Patrick VM. Positive mood and resistance to temptation: The interfering influence of elevated arousal. *J Consum Res.* 2010; 37(4): 698–711. DOI: 10.1086/655665.

Felger JC. Imaging the role of inflammation in mood and anxiety-related disorders. *Curr Neuropharmacol.* 2018; 16(5): 533–58. DOI:10.2174/1570159X15666171123201142.

Finassi CM, Calixto LA, Segura W, et al. Effect of sweetened beverages intake on salivary aspartame, insulin, and alpha-amylase levels: A single-blind study. *Food Res Int.* 2023; 173(2): 113406. DOI: 10.1016/j.foodres.2023.113406.

Gangwisch JE, Hale L, Garcia L, et al. High glycemic index diet as a risk factor for depression: analyses from the Women's Health Initiative. *Am J Clin Nutr.* 2015 Aug; 102(2): 454–63. DOI: 10.3945/ajcn.114.103846. Epub 2015 Jun 24. PMID: 26109579; PMCID: PMC4515860.

Hall KD, Ayuketah A, Brychta R, et al. Ultra-processed diets cause excess calorie intake and weight gain: An inpatient randomized controlled trial of ad libitum food intake. *Cell Metab.* 2019 Jul 2; 30(1): 67–77.e3. DOI: 10.1016/j.cmet.2019.05.008. Epub 2019 May 16. Erratum in: *Cell Metab.* 2019 Jul 2; 30(1): 226. Erratum in: *Cell Metab.* 2020 Oct 6; 32(4): 690. PMID: 31105044; PMCID: PMC7946062.

Kubota S, Liu Y, Iizuka K, et al. A review of recent findings on meal sequence: An attractive dietary approach to prevention and management of type 2 diabetes. *Nutrients.* 2020; 12(9): 2502. DOI: 10.3390/nu12092502.

Lee CH, Giuliani F. The role of inflammation in depression and fatigue. *Front Immunol.* 2019 Jul 19; 10: 1696. DOI: 10.3389/fimmu.2019.01696.

Lee SH, Moore LV, Park S, et al. Adults meeting fruit and vegetable intake recommendations—United States, 2019. *MMWR Morb Mortal Wkly Rep.* 2022; 71: 1–9. DOI: 10.15585/mmwr.mm7101a1.

Li J, Lee DH, Hu J, et al. Dietary inflammatory potential and risk of cardiovascular disease among men and women in the US. *J Am Coll Cardiol.* 2020 Nov 10; 76(19): 2181–93. DOI: 10.1016/j.jacc.2020.09.535. PMID: 33153576; PMCID: PMC7745775.

Liu X, Jin Z, Summers S, et al. Calorie restriction and calorie dilution have different impacts on body fat, metabolism, behavior, and hypothalamic gene expression. *Cell Rep.* 2022 May 17; 39(7):110835. DOI: 10.1016/j.celrep.2022.110835. PMID: 35584669.

Loucks EB, Kronish IM, Saadeh FB, et al. Adapted mindfulness training for interoception and adherence to the DASH diet: A phase 2 randomized clinical trial. *JAMA Netw Open.* 2023; 6(11): e2339243. DOI: 10.1001/jamanetworkopen.2023.39243.

Mansur RB, Brietzke E, McIntyre RS. Is there a "metabolic-mood syndrome"? A review of the relationship between obesity and mood disorders. *Neurosci Biobehav Rev.* 2015 May; 52: 89–104. DOI: 10.1016/j.neubiorev.2014.12.017. Epub 2015 Jan 8. PMID: 25579847.

Martínez-González MA, Montero P, Ruiz-Canela M, et al. Yearly attained adherence to Mediterranean diet and incidence of diabetes in a large randomized trial. *Cardiovasc Diabetol.* 2023; 22: 262. DOI: 10.1186/s12933-023-01994-2.

McElroy SL, Kotwal R, Malhotra S, et al. Are mood disorders and obesity related? A review for the mental health professional. *J Clin Psychiatry.* 2004 May; 65(5): 634–51, quiz on 730. DOI: 10.4088/jcp.v65n0507. PMID: 15163249.

Moieni M, Eisenberger NI. Effects of inflammation on social processes and implications for health. *Ann N Y Acad Sci.* 2018 Sep; 1428(1): 5–13. DOI: 10.1111/nyas.13864. Epub 2018 May 28. PMID: 29806109; PMCID: PMC6158086.

Mussell MP, Mitchell JE, Weller CL, et al. Onset of binge eating, dieting, obesity, and mood disorders among subjects seeking treatment for binge eating disorder. *Int J Eat Disord.* 1995 May; 17(4): 395–401. DOI: 10.1002/1098-108x(199505)17:4<395::aid-eat2260170412>3.0.co;2-i. PMID: 7620480.

Nitta A, Imai S, Kajiayama S, et al. Impact of dietitian-led nutrition therapy of food order on 5-year glycemic control in outpatients with type 2 diabetes at primary care clinic: Retrospective cohort study. *Nutrients.* 2022; 14(14): 2865. DOI: 10.3390/nu14142865.

Pourmotabbed A, Moradi S, Babaei A, et al. Food insecurity and mental health: A systematic review and meta-analysis. *Public Health Nutr.* 2020 Jul; 23(10): 1778–90. DOI: 10.1017/S136898001900435X. Epub 2020 Mar 16. Erratum in: *Public Health Nutr.* 2020 Jul; 23(10): 1854. PMID: 32174292.

Puhl R, Brownell K. Confronting and coping with weight stigma: An investigation of overweight and obese adults. *Obesity.* 2006 Oct; 14(10): 1802–15. DOI: 10.1038/oby.2006.208.

Sánchez-Villegas A, Zazpe I, Santiago S, et al. Added sugars and sugar-sweetened beverage consumption, dietary carbohydrate index and depression risk in the Seguimiento Universidad de Navarra (SUN) Project. *Br J Nutr.* 2018 Jan; 119(2): 211–21. DOI: 10.1017/S0007114517003361. Epub 2017 Dec 22. PMID: 29268815.

Singh M. Mood, food, and obesity. *Front Psychol.* 2014 Sep 1; 5: 925. DOI: 10.3389/fpsyg.2014.00925.

Szuhany KL, Bugatti M, Otto MW. A meta-analytic review of the effects of exercise on brain-derived neurotrophic factor. *J Psychiatr Res.* 2015; 60: 56–64. DOI: 10.1016/j.jpsychires.2014.10.003.

CHAPTER 5: Nutrients

Appleton KM, Voyias PD, Sallis HM, et al. Omega-3 fatty acids for depression in adults. *Cochrane Database Syst Rev.* 2021 Nov; 11: CD004692. DOI: 10.1002/14651858 .CD004692.pub5.

Bakoyiannis J, Daskalopoulou A, Pergialiotis V, et al. Phytochemicals and cognitive health: Are flavonoids doing the trick? *Biomed Pharmacother.* 2019; 109: 1488–97. DOI: 10.1016/j.biopha.2018.10.086.

Bastiaanssen TFS, Cowan CSM, Claesson MJ, et al. Making sense of . . . the microbiome in psychiatry. *Int J Neuropsychopharmacol.* 2019 Jan 1; 22(1): 37–52. DOI: 10.1093/ijnp/ pyy067. PMID: 30099552; PMCID: PMC6313131.

Begley A, Fisher I, Butcher L, et al. Determining the effectiveness of an adult food literacy program using a matched control group. *J Nutr Educ Behav.* 2023; 55(9): 659–66. DOI: 10.1016/j.jneb.2023.06.001.

Bhaswant M, Shanmugam DK, Miyazawa T, et al. Microgreens: A comprehensive review of bioactive molecules and health benefits. *Molecules.* 2023 Jan 15; 28(2): 867. DOI: 10.3390/ molecules28020867.

Bizzozero-Peroni B, Fernández-Rodríguez R, Martínez-Vizcaíno V, et al. Nut consumption is associated with a lower risk of depression in adults: A prospective analysis with data from the UK Biobank cohort. *Clin Nutr.* 2023 Sep; 42(9): 1728–36. DOI: 10.1016/j .clnu.2023.07.020.

Bongers P, Jansen A, Havermans R. Happy eating: The underestimated role of overeating in a positive mood. *Appetite.* 2013 Aug; 67: 74–80. DOI: 10.1016/j.appet.2013.03.017.

Bushman BJ, Dewall CN, Pond RS Jr, et al. Low glucose relates to greater aggression in married couples. *Proc Natl Acad Sci USA.* 2014 Apr 29; 111(17): 6254–57. DOI: 10.1073/ pnas.1400619111. Epub 2014 Apr 14. PMID: 24733932; PMCID: PMC4035998.

Buydens-Branchey L, Branchey M, Hibbeln JR. Associations between increases in plasma n-3 polyunsaturated fatty acids following supplementation and decreases in anger and anxiety in substance abusers. *Prog Neuropsychopharmacol Biol Psychiatry.* 2008 Feb; 32(2): 568–75. DOI: 10.1016/j.pnpbp.2007.10.020.

Campisi SC, Cost KT, Korczak DJ. Food intake reporting bias among adolescents with depression. *Eur J Clin Nutr.* 2021. DOI: 10.1038/s41430-021-01035-9.

Chauhan A, Chauhan V. Beneficial effects of walnuts on cognition and brain health. *Nutrients.* 2020 Feb; 12(2): 550. DOI: 10.3390/nu12020550.

Chang SC, Cassidy A, Willett WC, et al. Dietary flavonoid intake and risk of incident depression in midlife and older women. *Am J Clin Nutr.* 2016 Sep; 104(3): 704–14. DOI: 10.3945/ajcn.115.124545.

Chintala SC, Liaukonyte J, Yang N. Browsing the aisles or browsing the app? How online grocery shopping is changing what we buy. *Marketing Science* (Articles in Advance). Published online August 2023: 1–17. DOI: 10.1287/mksc.2022.0292.

Conner TS, Brookie KL, Carr AQ, et al. Let them eat fruit! The effect of fruit and vegetable consumption on psychological well-being in young adults: A randomized controlled trial. *PLoS One.* 2017; 12(2): e0171206. DOI: 10.1371/journal.pone.0171206.

Crespo-Bujosa H, Gonzalez M, Duconge J, et al. Nutrient depletion-induced neuro-chemical disorder (brain hunger) as the basis of psychopathology and aggressive behavior. *J Orthomol Med.* 2017; 32.

Deuman KA, Callahan EA, Wang L, et al. *True Cost of Food: Food Is Medicine Case Study.* Food Is Medicine Institute, Friedman School, Tufts University. 2023.

Dowlati Y, Ravindran AV, Segal ZV, et al. Selective dietary supplementation in early postpartum is associated with high resilience against depressed mood. *Proc Natl Acad Sci USA.* 2017 Mar; 114(13): 3509–14. DOI: 10.1073/pnas.1611965114.

Downer S, Clippinger E, Kummer C. *Food is Medicine Research Action Plan.* Published 2022 Jan 27. Aspen Institute and Center for Health Law and Policy Innovation at Harvard Law School.

Finkel MA, Barrios D, Partida I, et al. Participant and stakeholder perceptions of the Food FARMacy emergency food assistance program for COVID-19: A qualitative study. *J Acad Nutr Diet.* 2023. DOI: 10.1016/j.jand.2023.10.021.

Folta SC, Li Z, Cash SB, et al. Adoption and implementation of produce prescription programs for under-resourced populations: Clinic staff perspectives. *Front Nutr.* 2023; 10: 1221785. DOI: 10.3389/fnut.2023.1221785.

Garfinkel SN, Zorab E, Navaratnam N, et al. Anger in brain and body: The neural and physiological perturbation of decision-making by emotion. *Soc Cogn Affect Neurosci.* 2016 Jan; 11(1): 150–58. DOI: 10.1093/scan/nsv099. Epub 2015 Aug 7. PMID: 26253525; PMCID: PMC4692323.

Gearhardt AN, Bueno NB, DiFeliceantonio AG, et al. Social, clinical, and policy implications of ultra-processed food addiction. *BMJ.* 2023; 383: e075354. DOI: 10.1136/bmj-2023-075354.

Golomb BA, Evans MA, White HL, et al. Trans fat consumption and aggression. *PLoS One.* 2012; 7(3): e32175. DOI: 10.1371/journal.pone.0032175. Epub 2012 Mar 5. PMID: 22403632; PMCID: PMC3293881.

Grosso G, Galvano F, Marventano S, et al. Omega-3 fatty acids and depression: Scientific evidence and biological mechanisms. *Oxid Med Cell Longev.* 2014; 2014: 313570. DOI: 10.1155/2014/313570.

Hamner HC, Dooyema CA, Blanck HM, et al. Fruit, vegetable, and sugar-sweetened beverage intake among young children, by state—United States, 2021. *MMWR Morb Mortal Wkly Rep.* 2023; 72:165–70. DOI: 10.15585/mmwr.mm7207a1.

Hibbeln JR, Ferguson TA, Blasbalg, TL. Omega-3 deficiencies in neurodevelopment, aggression, and autonomic dysregulation: opportunities for intervention. *International Review of Psychiatry.* 2006 Apr; 18(2): 107–18. DOI: 10.1080/09540260600582967.

Hillmire MR, DeVylder JE, Forestell CA. Fermented foods, neuroticism, and social anxiety: An interactive model. *Psychiatry Res.* 2015 Aug; 228(2): 203–8. DOI: 10.1016/j.psychres.2015.04.023.

Hollinger D. *Anatomy of Grief.* Yale University Press. 2020.

Huang S, Riccardi D, Pflanzer S, et al. Survivors Overcoming and Achieving Resiliency (SOAR): Mindful eating practice for breast cancer survivors in a virtual teaching kitchen. *Nutrients.* 2023; 15(19): 4205. DOI: 10.3390/nu15194205.

Huda MN, Lu S, Jahan T, et al. Treasure from garden: Bioactive compounds of buckwheat. *Food Chem.* 2021; 335: 127653. DOI: 10.1016/j.foodchem.2020.127653.

Jahangard L, Hedayati M, Abbasalipourkabir R, et al. Omega-3 polyunsaturated fatty acids (O3PUFAs), compared to placebo, reduced symptoms of occupational burnout and lowered morning cortisol secretion. *Psychoneuroendocrinology.* 2019 Nov; 109: 104384. DOI: 10.1016/j.psyneuen.2019.104384.

Jahangard L, Sadeghi A, Ahmadpanah M, et al. Influence of adjuvant omega-3 polyunsaturated fatty acids on depression, sleep, and emotion regulation among outpatients with major depressive orders-results from a double-blind, randomized and placebo-controlled clinical trial. *J Psychiatr Res.* 2018 Oct; 107: 48–56. DOI: 10.1016/j.jpsychires.2018.09.016.

Jónasdóttir, SH. Fatty acid profiles and production in marine phytoplankton. *Mar Drugs.* 2019; 17(3): 151. DOI: 10.3390/md17030151.

Kang JX. Omega-3: A link between global climate change and human health. *Biotechnol Adv.* 2011 Jul–Aug; 29(4): 388–90. DOI: 10.1016/j.biotechadv.2011.02.003. Epub 2011 Mar 23. PMID: 21406222; PMCID: PMC3090543.

Kennedy DO. B vitamins and the brain: Mechanisms, dose, and efficacy—A review. *Nutrients.* 2016 Jan; 8(2): 68. DOI: 10.3390/nu8020068.

Kiecolt-Glaser J, Belury MA, Andridge R, et al. Omega-3 supplementation lowers inflammation and anxiety in medical students: A randomized controlled trial. *Brain Behav Immun.* 2011; 25(8): 1725–34. DOI: 10.1016/j.bbi.2011.07.229.

Kim Y, Roberts AL, Rimm EB, et al. Posttraumatic stress disorder and changes in diet quality over 20 years among US women. *Psychol Med.* 2021; 51(2): 310–19. DOI: 10.1017/S0033291719003246.

Lam MHB, Chau SWH, Wing YK. High prevalence of hypokalemia in acute psychiatric patients. *Gen Hosp Psych.* 2009; 31(3): 262–65.

Larrieu T, Layé S. Food for mood: Relevance of nutritional omega-3 fatty acids for depression and anxiety. *Front Physiol.* 2018; 9: 1047. DOI: 10.3389/fphys.2018.01047.

Li J, Lee DH, Hu J, et al. Dietary inflammatory potential and risk of cardiovascular disease among men and women. *J Am Coll Cardiol.* 2020; 76(19): 2181–93. DOI: 10.1016/j.jacc.2020.09.535.

Liao Y, Xie B, Zhang H, et al. Efficacy of omega-3 PUFAs in depression: A meta-analysis. *Transl Psychiatry.* 2019; 9: 190. DOI: 10.1038/s41398-019-0515-5.

Logan AC. Omega-3 fatty acids and major depression: A primer for the mental health professional. *Lipids Health Dis.* 2004; 3: 25. DOI:10.1186/1476-511X-3-25.

Loucks EB, Kronish IM, Saadeh FB, et al. Adapted mindfulness training for interoception and adherence to the DASH diet: A phase 2 randomized clinical trial. *JAMA Netw Open.* 2023; 6(11): e2339243. DOI: 10.1001/jamanetworkopen.2023.39243.

Magnusson A, Axelsson J, Karlsson MM, Oskarsson H. Lack of seasonal mood change in the Icelandic population: Results of a cross-sectional study. *Am J Psychiatry*. 2000; 157(2): 234–38. DOI: 10.1176/appi.ajp.157.2.234.

Maqbool A, Strandvik B, Stallings V. The skinny on tuna fat: Health implications." *Public Health Nutr*. 2011 Nov; 14(11): 2049–54. DOI: 10.1017/S1368980010003757.

Masana MF, Tyrovolas S, Kolia N, et al. Dietary patterns and their association with anxiety symptoms among older adults: The ATTICA study. *Nutrients*. 2019 May 31; 11(6): 1250. DOI: 10.3390/nu11061250. PMID: 31159322; PMCID: PMC6627391.

Mathur M, Marshall A, Yeragi P, et al. Design and protocol of a clinic-based comparative effectiveness randomized controlled trial to determine the feasibility and effectiveness of food prescription program strategies in at-risk pediatric populations. *Contemp Clin Trials*. 2023; 135: 107379. DOI: 10.1016/j.cct.2023.107379.

Mihrshahi S, Dobson A, Mishra G. Fruit and vegetable consumption and prevalence and incidence of depressive symptoms in mid-age women: Results from the Australian longitudinal study on women's health. *Eur J Clin Nutr*. 2015; 69: 585–91. DOI: 10.1038/ejcn.2014.222.

Mocking RJT, Harmsen I, Assies J, et al. Meta-analysis and meta-regression of omega-3 polyunsaturated fatty acid supplementation for major depressive disorder. *Transl Psychiatry*. 2016 Mar; 6(3): e756. DOI: 10.1038/tp.2016.29.

Monteiro CA, Cannon G, Lawrence M, et al. *Ultra-processed foods, diet quality, and health using the NOVA classification system*. Rome: FAO. 2019.

Mostofsky E, Penner EA, Mittleman MA. Outbursts of anger as a trigger of acute cardiovascular events: A systematic review and meta-analysis. *Eur Heart J*. 2014 Jun 1; 35(21): 1404–10. DOI: 10.1093/eurheartj/ehu033. Epub 2014 Mar 3. PMID: 24591550; PMCID: PMC4043318.

Mujcic R, Oswald AJ. Evolution of well-being and happiness after increases in consumption of fruit and vegetables. *Am J Public Health*. 2016 Aug; 106(8): 1504–10.

O'Connor LE, Hall KD, Zhang FF, et al. A research roadmap about ultra-processed foods and human health for the United States food system: Proceedings from an interdisciplinary, multi-stakeholder workshop (Perspective). *Adv Nutr*. 2023; 14(6): 1255–69. DOI: 10.1016/j.advnut.2023.09.005.

Pang B, Memel Z, Diamant C, et al. Culinary medicine and community partnership: Hands-on culinary skills training to empower medical students to provide patient-centered nutrition education. *Med Educ Online*. 2019; 24(1): 1630238. DOI: 10.1080/10872981.2019.1630238.

Papandreou C. Independent associations between fatty acids and sleep quality among obese patients with obstructive sleep apnoea syndrome. *J Sleep Res*. 2013 Oct; 22(5): 569–72. DOI: 10.1111/jsr.12043.

Peltomaa E, Johnson MD, Taipale SJ. Marine cryptophytes are great sources of EPA DHA. *Mar Drugs*. 2018 Jan; 16(1): 3. DOI: 10.3390/md16010003.

Rees J, Bagatini SR, Lo J, et al. Association between fruit and vegetable intakes and mental health in the Australian diabetes obesity and lifestyle cohort. *Nutrients*. 2021 Apr; 13(5): 1447. DOI: 10.3390/nu13051447.

Reyes-Mendez ME, Castro-Sánchez LA, Dagnino-Acosta A, et al. Capsaicin produces antidepressant-like effects in the forced swimming test and enhances the response of a sub-effective dose of amitriptyline in rats. *Physiol Behav.* 2018 Oct 15; 195:158–66. DOI: 10.1016/j.physbeh.2018.08.006. Epub 2018 Aug 20. PMID: 30138635.

Samuthpongtorn C, Nguyen LH, Okereke OI, et al. Consumption of ultraprocessed food and risk of depression. *JAMA Netw Open.* 2023; 6(9): e2334770. DOI: 10.1001/jamanetworkopen.2023.34770.

Sastre LR, Stroud B, and Haldeman L. Simple but tailored: Developing culinary-focused nutrition education along with a produce prescription program. *J Nutr Educ Behav.* GEM No. 621. 2023; 55(11); P841–45. DOI: 10.1016/j.jneb.2023.07.013.

Scalbert A, Johnson IT, Saltmarsh M. Polyphenols: Antioxidants and beyond. *Am J Clin Nutr.* 2005 Jan; 81(1 Suppl): 215S–217S. DOI: 10.1093/ajcn/81.1.215S. PMID: 15640483.

Shelton RC, Manning JS, Barrentine LW, et al. Assessing effects of l-methylfolate in depression management: Results of a real-world patient experience trial. *Prim Care Companion CNS Discord.* 2013; 15(4): PCC.13m01520. DOI: 10.4088/PCC.13m01520.

Stroud B, Jacobs MM, Palakshappa D, et al. A rural delivery-based produce prescription intervention improves glycemic control and stress. *J Nutr Educ Behav.* 2023; 55(11): 803–14. DOI: 10.1016/j.jneb.2023.08.006.

Su KP, Matsuoka Y, Pae CU. Omega-3 polyunsaturated fatty acids in prevention of mood and anxiety disorders. *Clin Psychopharmacol Neurosci.* 2015 Aug; 13(2): 129–37. DOI: 10.9758/cpn.2015.13.2.129.

Su KP, Tseng PT, Lin PY, et al. Association of use of omega-3 polyunsaturated fatty acids with changes in severity of anxiety symptoms. *JAMA Netw Open.* 2018; 1(5): e182327. DOI: 10.1001/jamanetworkopen.2018.2327.

Tangney CC, Aggarwal NT, Li H, et al. Vitamin B$_{12}$, cognition, and brain MRI measures: A cross-sectional examination. *Neurology.* 2011 Sep; 77(13): 1276–82. DOI: 10.1212/WNL.0b013e3182315a33.

Vaidyanathan G. Healthy diets for people and the planet. *Nature.* 2021 Dec; 600: 22–25.

Wallace CJK, Milev R. The effects of probiotics on depressive symptoms in humans: A systematic review. *Annals of General Psychiatry.* 2017; 16(14). DOI: 10.1186/s12991-017-0138-2.

Wang A, Wan X, Zhuang P, et al. High fried food consumption impacts anxiety and depression due to lipid metabolism disturbance and neuroinflammation. *Proc Natl Acad Sci USA.* 2023 May 2; 120(18): e2221097120. DOI: 10.1073/pnas.2221097120.

White BA, Horwath CC, Conner TS. Many apples a day keep the blues away: Daily experience of negative and positive affect and food consumption in young adults. *Br J Health Psych.* 2013 Jan; 18(4): 782–98. DOI: 10.1111/bjhp.12021.

Williams JE, Paton CC, Siegler IC, et al. Anger proneness predicts coronary heart disease risk: Prospective analysis from the atherosclerosis risk in communities (ARIC) study. *Circulation.* 2000 May 2; 101(17): 2034–39. DOI: 10.1161/01.cir.101.17.2034. PMID: 10790343.

Xu Y, Wang C, Klabnik JJ, et al. Novel therapeutic targets in depression and anxiety: Antioxidants as a candidate for treatment. *Current Neuropharmacology.* 2014; 12(2): 108–19. DOI: 10.2174/1570159X11666131120231448.

Yoshikawa E, Nishi D, Matsuoka YJ. Association between frequency of fried food consumption and resilience to depression in Japanese company workers: A cross-sectional study. *Lipids Health Dis.* 2016 Sep 15; 15(1): 156. DOI: 10.1186/s12944-016-0331-3.

Recipe Index

Index

About the Author

MARY BETH ALBRIGHT is a writer, editor, and
executive producer at the *Washington Post*. She has
worked at the US Surgeon General's office and
written for *National Geographic*, appeared on the
Food Network, and earned degrees from Johns
Hopkins and Georgetown. She lives in Washington, DC, with her son.